Comparative Effectiveness Review
Number 105

Interventions To Improve Cardiovascular Risk Factors in People With Serious Mental Illness

Prepared for:
Agency for Healthcare Research and Quality
U.S. Department of Health and Human Services
540 Gaither Road
Rockville, MD 20850
www.ahrq.gov

Contract No. 290-2007-10066-I

Prepared by:
Duke Evidence-based Practice Center
Durham, NC

Investigators:
Jennifer M. Gierisch, Ph.D., M.P.H.
Jason A. Nieuwsma, Ph.D.
Daniel W. Bradford, M.D., M.P.H.
Christine M. Wilder, M.D.
Monica C. Mann-Wrobel, Ph.D.
Amanda J. McBroom, Ph.D.
Liz Wing, M.A.
Michael D. Musty, B.A.
Megan M. Chobot, M.S.L.S.
Vic Hasselblad, Ph.D.
John W. Williams, Jr., M.D., M.H.Sc.

AHRQ Publication No. 13-EHC063-EF
April 2013

This report is based on research conducted by the Duke Evidence-based Practice Center (EPC) under contract to the Agency for Healthcare Research and Quality (AHRQ), Rockville, MD (Contract No. 290-2007-10066-I). The findings and conclusions in this document are those of the authors, who are responsible for its contents; the findings and conclusions do not necessarily represent the views of AHRQ. Therefore, no statement in this report should be construed as an official position of AHRQ or of the U.S. Department of Health and Human Services.

The information in this report is intended to help health care decisionmakers—patients and clinicians, health system leaders, and policymakers, among others—make well-informed decisions and thereby improve the quality of health care services. This report is not intended to be a substitute for the application of clinical judgment. Anyone who makes decisions concerning the provision of clinical care should consider this report in the same way as any medical reference and in conjunction with all other pertinent information, i.e., in the context of available resources and circumstances presented by individual patients.

This report may be used, in whole or in part, as the basis for development of clinical practice guidelines and other quality enhancement tools, or as a basis for reimbursement and coverage policies. AHRQ or U.S. Department of Health and Human Services endorsement of such derivative products may not be stated or implied.

This document is in the public domain and may be used and reprinted without permission except those copyrighted materials that are clearly noted in the document. Further reproduction of those copyrighted materials is prohibited without the specific permission of copyright holders.

Persons using assistive technology may not be able to fully access information in this report. For assistance contact EffectiveHealthCare@ahrq.hhs.gov.

Suggested citation: Gierisch JM, Nieuwsma JA, Bradford DW, Wilder CM, Mann-Wrobel MC, McBroom AJ, Wing L, Musty MD, Chobot MM, Hasselblad V, Williams JW Jr. Interventions To Improve Cardiovascular Risk Factors in People With Serious Mental Illness. Comparative Effectiveness Review No. 105. (Prepared by the Duke Evidence-based Practice Center under Contract No. 290-2007-10066-I.) AHRQ Publication No. 13-EHC063-EF. Rockville, MD: Agency for Healthcare Research and Quality. April 2013. www.effectivehealthcare.ahrq.gov/reports/final.cfm.

Preface

The Agency for Healthcare Research and Quality (AHRQ), through its Evidence-based Practice Centers (EPCs), sponsors the development of systematic reviews to assist public- and private-sector organizations in their efforts to improve the quality of health care in the United States. These reviews provide comprehensive, science-based information on common, costly medical conditions, and new health care technologies and strategies.

Systematic reviews are the building blocks underlying evidence-based practice; they focus attention on the strength and limits of evidence from research studies about the effectiveness and safety of a clinical intervention. In the context of developing recommendations for practice, systematic reviews can help clarify whether assertions about the value of the intervention are based on strong evidence from clinical studies. For more information about AHRQ EPC systematic reviews, see www.effectivehealthcare.ahrq.gov/reference/purpose.cfm

AHRQ expects that these systematic reviews will be helpful to health plans, providers, purchasers, government programs, and the health care system as a whole. Transparency and stakeholder input are essential to the Effective Health Care Program. Please visit the Web site (www.effectivehealthcare.ahrq.gov) to see draft research questions and reports or to join an email list to learn about new program products and opportunities for input.

We welcome comments on this systematic review. They may be sent by mail to the Task Order Officer named below at: Agency for Healthcare Research and Quality, 540 Gaither Road, Rockville, MD 20850, or by email to epc@ahrq.hhs.gov.

Carolyn M. Clancy, M.D.
Director
Agency for Healthcare Research and Quality

Jean Slutsky, P.A., M.S.P.H.
Director, Center for Outcomes and Evidence
Agency for Healthcare Research and Quality

Stephanie Chang M.D., M.P.H.
Director, EPC Program
Center for Outcomes and Evidence
Agency for Healthcare Research and Quality

Marian James, M.D.
Task Order Officer
Center for Outcomes and Evidence
Agency for Healthcare Research and Quality

Acknowledgments

The authors thank Megan von Isenburg, M.S.L.S., for help with the literature search and retrieval.

Key Informants

Christine Collins, M.S.W.
Deputy Director
North Carolina Office of Rural Health and
  Community Care
Raleigh, NC

Benjamin G. Druss, M.D., M.P.H.
Professor, Rollins School of Public Health
Emory University
Atlanta, GA

Laura J. Fochtmann, M.D.
Professor of Psychiatry
Stony Brook University
Stony Brook, NY

Parinda Khatri, Ph.D.
Clinical Psychologist
Cherokee Health Systems
Knoxville, TN

Amy M. Kilbourne, Ph.D., M.P.H.
Associate Professor of Psychiatry
University of Michigan
Ann Arbor, MI

Michael Weaver, M.S.Ed.
Executive Director
Mental Health America of the Tar River
  Region
Rocky Mount, NC

Judy Zerzan, M.D., M.P.H.
Colorado Medicaid Medical Director
Colorado Department of Health Care Policy
  and Financing
Denver, CO

Technical Expert Panel

Christine Collins, M.S.W.
Deputy Director
North Carolina Office of Rural Health and
  Community Care
Raleigh, NC

Lisa M. Dixon, M.D., M.P.H
Director, Center for Practice Innovations
New York State Psychiatric Institute
New York, NY

Benjamin G. Druss, M.D., M.P.H.
Professor, Rollins School of Public Health
Emory University
Atlanta, GA

Laura J. Fochtmann, M.D.
Professor of Psychiatry
Stony Brook University
Stony Brook, NY

Martha Gerrity, M.D., M.P.H. Ph.D.
Clinical Evidence Specialty
Oregon Health & Science University
Portland, OR

Louise M. Howard, Ph.D.
Professor in Women's Mental Health
King's College London
London, UK

Amy M. Kilbourne, Ph.D., M.P.H.
Associate Professor of Psychiatry
University of Michigan
Ann Arbor, MI

Anthony F. Lehman, M.D., M.S.P.H.
Professor of Psychiatry
University of Maryland
Baltimore, MD

T. Scott Stroup, M.D., M.P.H.
Professor of Psychiatry
Columbia University
New York, NY

Alexander S. Young, M.D., M.S.H.S
Professor of Psychiatry
University of California, Los Angeles
Los Angeles, CA

Peer Reviewers

Stephen J. Bartels, M.D., M.S.
Professor of Psychiatry
The Dartmouth Institute for Health Police &
  Clinical Research
Lebanon, NH

Amy N. Cohen, Ph.D.
Professor of Psychology
University of California, Los Angeles
Los Angeles, CA

Gerald Gartlehner, M.D., M.P.H.
Department Head, Evidence-based Medicine
  and Clinical Epidemiology
Danube University
Krems, Austria

Julie A. Kreyenbuhl, Pharm.D., Ph.D.
Associate Professor of Psychiatry
University of Maryland
Baltimore, MD

Paul Pirraglia, M.D.
Assistant Professor of Medicine
Brown University
Providence, RI

Andrew M. Pomerantz, Ph.D.
Professor of Psychology
Southern Illinois University
Edwardsville, IL

Martha Sajatovic, M.D.
Professor of Psychiatry
University Hospitals of Cleveland
Cleveland, OH

Interventions To Improve Cardiovascular Risk Factors in People With Serious Mental Illness

Structured Abstract

Objectives. Individuals with serious mental illness (SMI) have excess mortality from cardiovascular disease (CVD) and high rates of CVD risk factors such as diabetes, obesity, and hyperlipidemia. We conducted a systematic review to evaluate interventions to improve CVD risk factors in adults with SMI.

Data Sources. We searched PubMed[®], Embase[®], PsycINFO[®], and the Cochrane Database of Systematic Reviews for English-language trials published since 1980 that evaluated patient-focused behavioral interventions, peer or family support interventions, pharmacological treatments, and multicondition lifestyle interventions, or their combination, that targeted weight control, glucose levels, lipid levels, or CVD risk profile among adults with SMI at elevated risk of CVD.

Review Methods. Two investigators screened each abstract and full-text article for inclusion, abstracted data, and performed quality ratings, efficacy–effectiveness ratings, and evidence grading. Qualitative and quantitative methods, using random-effects models, were used to summarize results.

Results. Of 35 eligible studies, most enrolled patients with schizophrenia who were prescribed antipsychotics. Most studies were designed to control weight (n=28); one study specifically addressed diabetes management, none targeted hyperlipidemia, and three were multicondition interventions. Most studies were efficacy trials comparing behavioral interventions with control; none evaluated peer and family support. There were few direct comparisons of active interventions; effects on overall CVD risk, physical functioning, or cardiovascular events were reported rarely.

Compared with controls, behavioral interventions (mean difference [MD] -3.13 kg; 95% CI, -4.21 to -2.05), metformin (MD -4.13 kg; CI, -6.58 to -1.68), the anticonvulsive medications topiramate and zonisamide (MD -5.11kg; CI, -9.48 to -0.74), and adjunctive or antipsychotic switching to aripiprazole improved weight control. However, aripiprazole switching may be associated with higher rates of treatment failure. Nizatidine did not improve any outcome. The evidence was insufficient for all other interventions and effects on glucose and lipid control.

Conclusions. Few studies have evaluated interventions to address one or more CVD risk factors in patients with SMI. Comparative effectiveness studies are needed to test multimodal strategies, agents known to be effective in non-SMI populations, and antipsychotic-management strategies.

Contents

Executive Summary ES-1

Introduction 1
  Background 1
    Serious Mental Illness and Cardiovascular Health 1
    Current Treatment Approaches 2
  Scope and Key Questions 3
    Scope of the Review 3
    Key Questions 4
    Analytic Framework 5
  Organization of This Report 6

Methods 7
  Topic Refinement and Review Protocol 7
  Literature Search Strategy 7
    Sources Searched 7
    Inclusion and Exclusion Criteria 8
    Study Selection 10
  Data Extraction 10
  Quality Assessment of Individual Studies 11
  Data Synthesis 12
  Strength of the Body of Evidence 13
  Applicability 14
  Peer Review and Public Commentary 14

Results 15
  Introduction 15
  Results of Literature Searches 15
  Description of Included Studies 17
    Treatment Network Map 17
    Drugs Evaluated 19
    Efficacy–Effectiveness Scale 20
  Key Question 1. Effectiveness of Weight-Management Interventions 21
    Key Points 21
    Detailed Synthesis 22
    Summary of Key Question 1 32
  Key Question 2. Effectiveness of Diabetes-Management Interventions 33
    Key Points 33
    Detailed Synthesis 33
    Summary of Key Question 2 38
  Key Question 3. Effectiveness of Dyslipidemia-Management Interventions 39
    Key Points 39
    Detailed Synthesis 39
    Summary of Key Question 3 45
  Key Question 4. Effectiveness of Multicondition Lifestyle Interventions 45
    Key Points 45
    Detailed Synthesis 46
    Summary of Key Question 4 49

Discussion..51
    Key Findings and Strength of Evidence 51
        Key Question 1: Weight Control 52
        Key Question 2: Diabetes Control 54
        Key Question 3: Lipid Control 55
        Key Question 4: Multicondition Lifestyle Interventions 57
    Findings in Relation to What Is Already Known...59
    Applicability 58
    Implications for Clinical and Policy Decisionmaking 59
    Limitations of the Comparative Effectiveness Review Process 61
    Research Gaps..61
    Conclusions...64
References 65
Abbreviations 75

Tables
Table A. Overview of treatment effects and SOE by intervention and major outcomes........ ES-13
Table B. Evidence gaps and future research for adults with SMI ES-17
Table 1. Selected pharmacological treatments and behavioral strategies to manage
    CVD risk factors 3
Table 2. Inclusion and exclusion criteria 8
Table 3. Definitions of overall quality ratings 12
Table 4. Strength of evidence required domains 13
Table 5. Drugs evaluated 19
Table 6. Study characteristics for KQ 1: Weight-management interventions 23
Table 7. Details of behavioral interventions 24
Table 8. Study characteristics for KQ 2: Diabetes-management interventions..................... 34
Table 9. Study characteristics for KQ 3: Dyslipidemia-management interventions 41
Table 10. Study characteristics for KQ 4: Multicondition lifestyle interventions..................... 47
Table 11. Overview of treatment effects and SOE by intervention and major outcomes 51
Table 12. Summary SOE for KQ 1: Interventions for weight control............................ 53
Table 13. Summary SOE for KQ 2: Interventions for diabetes control (glucose)....................... 55
Table 14. Summary SOE for KQ 3: Interventions for lipid control 56
Table 15. Summary SOE for KQ 4: Multicondition lifestyle interventions............................. 57
Table 16. Evidence gaps and future research for adults with SMI   63

Figures
Figure A. Analytic framework.. ES-3
Figure B. Literature flow diagram ES-8
Figure 1. Analytic framework.. 5
Figure 2. Literature flow diagram.. 16
Figure 3. Treatment network describing the number of comparisons for each
    intervention (35 trials).. 18
Figure 4. Proportion of studies rated as studies of effectiveness on each
    efficacy—effectiveness dimension 20
Figure 5. Forest plot of meta-analysis of effect of behavioral interventions on weight 26

Figure 6. Forest plot of meta-analysis of effect of anticonvulsant medications
      topiramate and zonisamide on weight.. 28
Figure 7. Forest plot of meta-analysis of effect of metformin on weight..................................... 29
Figure 8. Forest plot of meta-analysis of effect of nizatidine on weight 31
Figure 9. Forest plot of meta-analysis of effect of behavioral interventions on LDL levels........ 42

Appendixes
Appendix A. Exact Search Strings
Appendix B. Efficacy–Effectiveness Rating Form
Appendix C. Data Abstraction Elements
Appendix D. Included Studies
Appendix E. Excluded Studies
Appendix F. Study Characteristics Table

Executive Summary

Background

Serious mental illness (SMI) is defined generally as a major mental or behavioral disorder, causing substantial impairment in multiple areas of daily functioning. SMI affects about 4 to 8 percent of adults[1-3] and includes disorders such as schizophrenia and bipolar disorder but not isolated substance abuse or developmental disorders. Individuals with SMI have shortened life expectancies relative to the general population to an extent that is not explained by suicide and accidents alone.[4,5] This population experiences higher rates of morbidity from multiple general medical conditions, including diabetes[6-8] and cardiovascular disease (CVD).[9-11] Among patients using the public mental health system, heart disease was the leading cause of death.[12] This excess of CVD-related mortality may be due to a number of factors, including direct effects of the illness, medications used to treat SMI, modifiable behavioral risk factors, and disparities in access and quality of health care.

For CVD, mental illness may be an independent risk factor that acts both directly through physiological effects such as underlying genetic vulnerabilities, or indirectly through effects on an individual's access to or interaction with the health care system.[13-15] Modifiable CVD risk factors, such as smoking,[16] obesity,[17,18] and physical inactivity[19,20] are highly prevalent among adults with SMI. Adverse effects of psychotropic drugs (notably second-generation antipsychotics) also may contribute to the development of CVD by increasing the risk of conditions such as hyperglycemia, hyperlipidemia, and obesity.[21] Lower socioeconomic status is more common in individuals with SMI[22,23] and may limit access to healthy food, opportunities for physical exercise (e.g., walkable neighborhoods and access to fitness facilities), and high-quality medical care. Numerous studies have demonstrated disparities in the quality of general medical care provided to individuals with SMI.[24-28] In contrast to individuals with less severe mental disorders, who largely receive mental health treatment in primary care settings, most individuals with SMI receive mental health treatment in specialized mental health settings. Consequently, people with SMI receive fewer preventive medical services[24,25] and less frequent guideline-concordant treatment to manage chronic physical illnesses such as diabetes[26,27] and CVD.[28] Given these issues, identifying intervention strategies that address CVD risk in individuals with SMI is a pressing priority to avoid early morbidity and mortality.

Scope and Key Questions

This comparative effectiveness review was funded by the Agency for Healthcare Research and Quality (AHRQ). The review was designed to evaluate strategies to improve CVD risk factors in adults with SMI. SMI has been defined variously by different groups over time.[29] For the purposes of this evidence review, people with SMI are defined as individuals who have: (1) schizophrenia or schizoaffective disorder (or other related primary psychotic disorder), (2) bipolar disorder, or (3) current major depression with psychotic features. We also included studies that enrolled adults with SMI or severe and persistent mental illness (SPMI) but did not specify diagnoses. Individuals with a primary diagnosis of substance abuse, dementia, personality disorder, or mental retardation are excluded from this definition.

To prioritize interventions for review, we examined published systematic reviews of strategies to improve CVD risk factors in individuals with SMI and consulted with our Key Informants. Because we identified recent high-quality reviews of general health advice, interventions for smoking cessation, and models to provide integrated mental health–general medical care, we elected not to cover these interventions again in our review.[30-34] We included randomized controlled trials (RCTs) of the pharmacological and patient-focused behavioral strategies along with peer and family support interventions. For patient-level intervention strategies, RCTs yield the highest quality evidence. We included both active and control comparators. Major outcomes of interest for this report are primary CVD risk factors (excluding tobacco use, as explained above), physical functioning or health-related quality of life, adverse effects, and all-cause mortality.

Key Questions

With input from our Technical Expert Panel (TEP), we constructed Key Questions (KQs) using the general approach of specifying the population of interest, interventions, comparators, outcomes, timing of outcomes, and settings (PICOTS). The KQs considered in this comparative effectiveness review were:

KQ 1: What is the effectiveness of weight-management behavioral interventions (e.g., behavioral counseling, health education), peer or family support interventions, pharmacological treatments (e.g., orlistat, topiramate), antipsychotic medication--switching to an antipsychotic with a low or neutral impact on weight, or their combination on weight control and related physical health outcomes (e.g., health-related quality of life, mortality) compared with each other or with usual care (or other control) among adults with serious mental illness (SMI) who are overweight, obese, or taking antipsychotics?

KQ 2: What is the effectiveness of diabetes-management behavioral interventions (e.g., behavioral counseling, health education), peer or family support interventions, pharmacological treatments (e.g., rosiglitazone, metformin), antipsychotic medication–switching to an antipsychotic with a low or neutral impact on glucose level, or their combination on glucose-level control and related physical health outcomes (e.g., health-related quality of life, mortality) compared with each other or with usual care (or other control) among adults with SMI who have diabetes or are taking antipsychotics?

KQ 3: What is the effectiveness of dyslipidemia-management behavioral interventions (e.g., behavioral counseling, health education), peer or family support interventions, pharmacological treatments (e.g., statins), antipsychotic medication–switching to an antipsychotic with a low or neutral impact on lipid levels, or their combination on lipid-level control and related physical health outcomes (e.g., health-related quality of life, mortality) compared with each other or with usual care (or other control) among adults with SMI who have dyslipidemia or are taking antipsychotics?

KQ 4: What is the effectiveness of multicondition lifestyle interventions (e.g., combinations of smoking cessation, physical activity, and nutrition counseling with or without medication management) on cardiovascular risk factors and related physical health outcomes (e.g., health-related quality of life, mortality) among adults with SMI who have cardiovascular disease, elevated cardiovascular risk (e.g., hypertension), or are taking antipsychotics?

Analytic Framework

Figure A depicts the KQs in the context of the PICOTS.

Figure A. Analytic framework

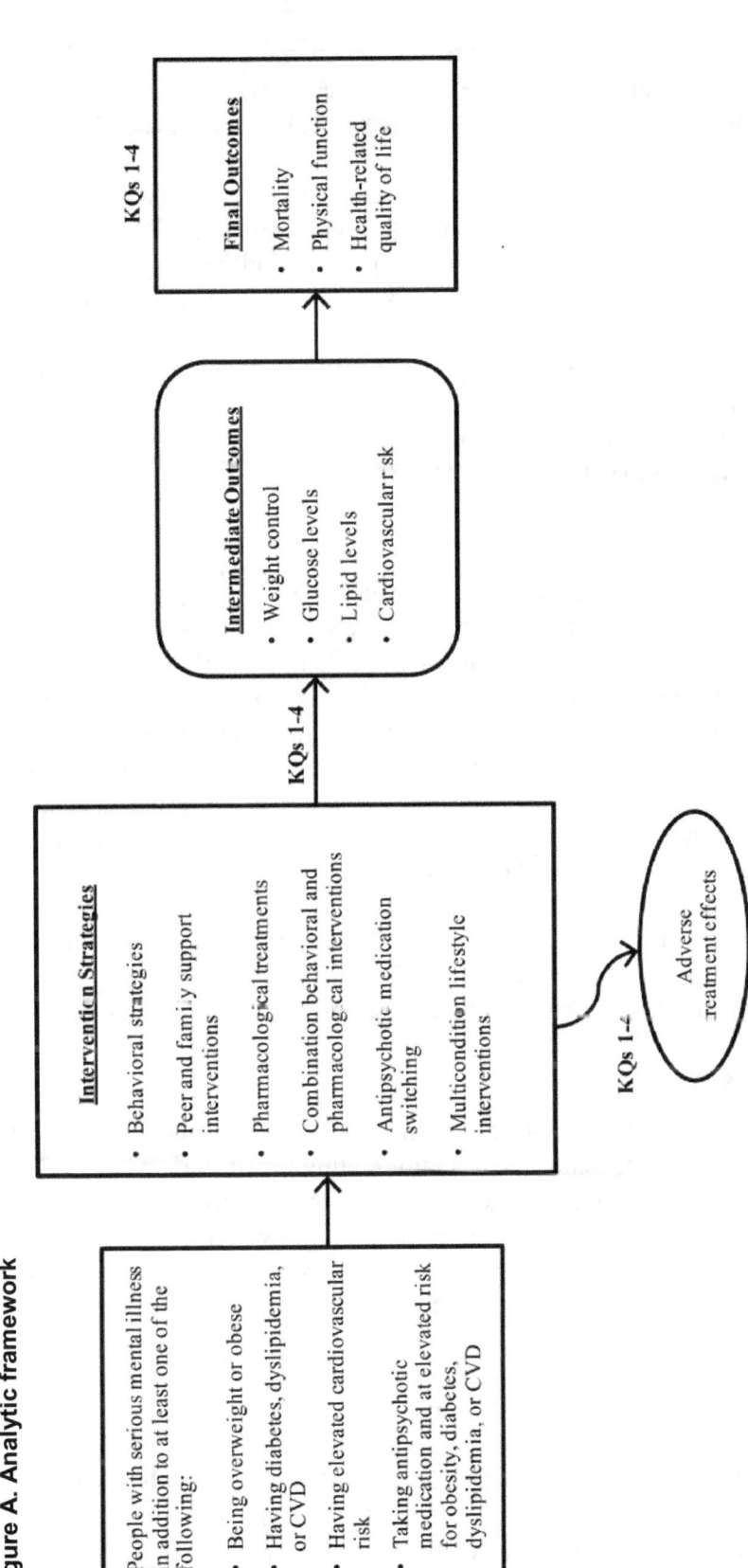

CVD = cardiovascular disease; KQ = Key Question

ES-3

Methods

The methods for this comparative effectiveness review follow those suggested in the AHRQ "Methods Guide for Effectiveness and Comparative Effectiveness Reviews" (available at www.effectivehealthcare.ahrq.gov/methodsguide.cfm; hereafter referred to as the Methods Guide).[35]

During the topic refinement stage, we solicited input from Key Informants representing clinicians, patient advocates, scientific experts, and payers to help define the Key Questions (KQs). The KQs were then posted for a 4-week public comment period, and the comments received were considered in the development of the research protocol. We next convened a TEP comprising clinical, content, and methodological experts to provide input in defining populations, interventions, comparisons, and outcomes, as well as identifying particular studies or databases to search. TEP members were invited to provide feedback on an initial draft of the review protocol, which was then refined based on their input, reviewed by AHRQ, and posted for public access at the AHRQ Effective Health Care Web site.[36]

Literature Search Strategy

To identify the relevant published literature, we searched MEDLINE®, Embase®, PsycINFO®, and the Cochrane Database of Systematic Reviews. Where possible, we used existing validated search filters (such as the Clinical Queries Filters in PubMed®). An experienced search librarian guided all searches. Exact search strings and dates are included in the appendix to the main report. We supplemented the electronic searches with a manual search of citations from a set of key primary and review articles. The reference lists for these articles were manually reviewed and cross-referenced against our library of search results, and additional potentially relevant citations were retrieved for screening. All citations were imported into an electronic database (EndNote® X4; Thomson Reuters, Philadelphia, PA).

We used two approaches to identify relevant gray literature: (1) a request for scientific information packets submitted to drug manufacturers and (2) a search of trial records listed in ClinicalTrials.gov. The search of ClinicalTrials.gov was also used as a mechanism to ascertain publication bias by identifying completed but unpublished studies.

Inclusion and Exclusion Criteria

Criteria used to screen articles for inclusion/exclusion at both the title-and-abstract and full-text screening stages are detailed in the main report. In brief, eligibility criteria were English-language RCTs that assess patient-focused behavioral interventions, peer or family support interventions, pharmacological treatments (including antipsychotic switching), multicondition lifestyle interventions, or their combination targeting weight control, glucose levels, lipid levels, or CVD risk profile among adults with SMI at elevated risk of CVD. We excluded articles describing studies that: (1) had as their primary goal improving psychiatric outcomes, (2) assessed only mass media strategies, (3) evaluated pharmacological agents not currently available on the U.S. market, or (4) took place in hospital or inpatient settings. Outcomes of interest were weight control (KQ 1); glucose level (i.e., hemoglobin A1c) (KQ 2); lipid level (i.e., change in low-density lipoprotein [LDL]) (KQ 3); CVD risk profile (e.g., Framingham CVD scores) or multiple individual components of modifiable CVD risk (e.g., lipid values, blood pressure, smoking status) (KQ 4); and health-related quality of life, all-cause mortality, physical function, serious adverse effects, and adverse effects (KQs 1–4).

Study Selection

Using the prespecified inclusion and exclusion criteria described in Table 2 of the full report, two investigators independently reviewed titles and abstracts for potential relevance to the KQs. Articles included by either reviewer underwent full-text screening. At the full-text screening stage, two investigators independently reviewed each article to determine if it met eligibility criteria, and indicated a decision to "include" or "exclude" the article for data abstraction. When the paired reviewers arrived at different decisions about whether to include or exclude an article, or about the reason for exclusion, they reconciled the difference through review and discussion, or through a third-party arbitrator if needed. Articles meeting our eligibility criteria were included for data abstraction. Relevant review articles and meta-analyses were flagged for manual searching of references and cross-referencing against the library of citations identified through electronic database searching. For citations retrieved by searching the gray literature, the above-described procedures were modified such that a single screener initially reviewed all search results; final eligibility of citations for data abstraction was determined by duplicate screening review. All screening decisions were made and tracked in a DistillerSR database (Evidence Partners Inc, Manotick, ON, Canada).

Data Extraction

The investigative team created data abstraction forms and evidence table templates for abstracting data for the KQs. Based on clinical and methodological expertise, a pair of investigators was assigned to abstract data from each eligible article. One investigator abstracted the data, and the second reviewed the article and the accompanying completed abstraction form to check for accuracy and completeness. Quality ratings and efficacy–effectiveness ratings (see below) were completed independently by two investigators. Disagreements were resolved by consensus, or by obtaining a third reviewer's opinion if consensus could not be reached. To aid in both reproducibility and standardization of data collection, researchers received data abstraction instructions directly on each form created specifically for this project within the DistillerSR database.

We designed the data abstraction forms for this project to collect the data required to evaluate the specified eligibility criteria for inclusion in this review, as well as demographic and other data needed for determining outcomes. We gave particular attention to describing the details of the interventions (e.g., pharmacotherapy used, intensity of behavioral interventions), patient characteristics (e.g., SMI diagnosis), and comparators that may be related to outcomes. Data necessary for assessing quality and applicability, as described in the Methods Guide,[35] were also abstracted. When critical data were missing, we contacted study authors. Of the seven authors contacted, five replied with the requested information.

Quality Assessment of Individual Studies

We evaluated the quality of individual studies using the key criteria for RCTs described in the Methods Guide.[35] Criteria of interest included methods of randomization and allocation concealment, similarity of groups at baseline, extent to which outcomes were described, blinding of subjects and providers, blinded assessment of the outcome(s), intention-to-treat analysis, differential loss to followup between the compared groups or overall high loss to followup, and conflicts of interest.

To indicate the summary judgment of the quality of the individual studies, we used the summary ratings of good, fair, or poor based on their adherence to well-accepted standard methodologies and adequate reporting. For each study, two investigators independently assigned a summary quality rating; disagreements were resolved by consensus or by discussion with a third investigator if agreement could not be reached. Quality ratings were assigned separately for "hard" outcomes (e.g., mortality, laboratory measurements) and all other outcomes (e.g., health-related quality of life); thus, a given study may have been categorized differently for two individual outcomes reported within that study.

Data Synthesis

We began by summarizing key features of the included studies for each Key Question. We then determined the feasibility of completing a quantitative synthesis (i.e., meta-analysis). Feasibility depended on the volume of relevant literature (≥ 3 studies), conceptual homogeneity of the studies, and completeness of the reporting of results. When a meta-analysis was appropriate, we used random-effects models to quantitatively synthesize the available evidence. For other outcomes we analyzed the results qualitatively. The outcomes amenable to meta-analysis were continuous; we therefore summarized these outcomes by a weighted difference of the means when the same scale (e.g., weight) was used and a standardized mean difference when the scales (e.g., health-related quality of life) differed across studies. We standardized results presentation such that a negative value indicates a greater intervention effect. We present summary estimates, standard errors, and confidence intervals in our data synthesis.

We organized our analyses by KQ. When a single study reported outcomes relevant to multiple KQs, it was included in the analyses for each question. For example, a study evaluating a weight-loss intervention that specified weight as the primary outcome—but also reported effects on glucose and lipid parameters—was described in each relevant KQ. When a study was designed to intervene on more than one CVD risk factor (e.g., metabolic syndrome), it was summarized in KQ 4. We specified, a priori, weight control as measured by change in kilograms (or pounds), hemoglobin A1c (HbA1c) as the preferred measure of glucose control since it reflects average glucose values over a 3-month interval, and total and LDL cholesterol as measures of lipid control. For adverse effects, we report significant worsening of psychiatric status and discontinuations due to adverse effects. Interventions were categorized as: behavioral, pharmacological, peer or family support, or multicondition (e.g., specifically targeting more than one condition such as smoking cessation and weight loss). Drug classes were psychotropics, neurologics, metformin, antihistamines, nutritionals (i.e., carnitine), and switching between antipsychotic medications.

We tested for heterogeneity using graphical displays and test statistics (Q statistic), while recognizing that the ability of statistical methods to detect heterogeneity may be limited.[37] The I^2 describes the percentage of total variation across studies due to heterogeneity rather than to chance. Heterogeneity was categorized as low, moderate, or high based on I^2 values of 25 percent, 50 percent, and 75 percent respectively.[37] All analyses were conducted using Comprehensive Meta-Analysis software (Version 2; Biostat, Englewood, NJ).

Strength of the Body of Evidence

The strength of evidence for each KQ and outcome was assessed using the approach described in the Methods Guide.[35,38] In brief, the approach requires assessment of four domains: risk of bias, consistency, directness, and precision. Additional domains were used when appropriate: coherence, and publication bias. These domains were considered qualitatively, and a summary rating of high, moderate, or low strength of evidence was assigned after discussion by two reviewers. In some cases, high, moderate, or low ratings were impossible or imprudent to make; for example, when no evidence was available or when evidence on the outcome was too weak, sparse, or inconsistent to permit any conclusion to be drawn. In these situations, a grade of insufficient was assigned.

Applicability

We assessed applicability across our KQs using the method described in the Methods Guide.[35,39] In brief, this method uses the PICOTS format as a way to organize information relevant to applicability. The most important issue with respect to applicability is whether the outcomes are different across studies that recruit different populations (e.g., age groups, exclusions for comorbidities) or use different methods to implement the interventions of interest; that is, important characteristics are those that affect baseline (control-group) rates of events, intervention-group rates of events, or both. We used a checklist to guide the assessment of applicability. We used these data to evaluate the applicability to clinical practice, paying special attention to study eligibility criteria, demographic features of the enrolled population in comparison with the target population, characteristics of the intervention used in comparison with care models currently in use, and clinical relevance and timing of the outcome measures. We summarized issues of applicability qualitatively.

Results

Figure B depicts the flow of articles through the literature search and screening process. Searches of PubMed®, Embase®, and the Cochrane Database of Systematic Reviews yielded 5,769 citations, 756 of which were duplicate citations. Manual searching identified 213 additional citations, for a total of 5,226 citations. After applying inclusion/exclusion criteria at the title-and-abstract level, 179 full-text articles were retrieved and screened. Of these, 139 were excluded at the full-text screening stage, leaving 40 articles (representing 35 unique studies) for data abstraction. No additional information was found through our gray literature search.

Overall, we included 35 studies, some of which were relevant to more than one KQ: 32 studies were relevant to KQ 1, 7 to KQ 2, 15 to KQ 3, and 3 to KQ 4. Studies were conducted in Europe (23%); Asia (14%); the United States (37%); Australia/New Zealand (6%); and South America (6%); or multiple continents (14%). Sixty-three percent of included studies enrolled individuals with schizophrenia or schizoaffective disorder, 11 percent recruited individuals with schizophrenia, schizoaffective disorder, or bipolar disorder, 20 percent recruited patients either taking antipsychotics or with an unspecified SMI diagnosis, and only 6 percent recruited individuals with bipolar disorder. The vast majority of studies were specifically designed to control weight (80%); only one study was designed to target diabetes management, and no studies were designed to target dyslipidemia.

The most common comparisons were between behavioral interventions and control (26% of comparisons), followed by neurologics (13%), and psychotropics or antihistamines compared with control (10% for each comparison). Relatively few studies compared two active interventions. No studies evaluated standard medications for hyperlipidemia (e.g., HMG-CoA reductase inhibitors) or orlistat (a Food and Drug Administration [FDA]-approved medication for weight control), and only a few studies evaluated hypoglycemic medication.

Figure B. Literature flow diagram

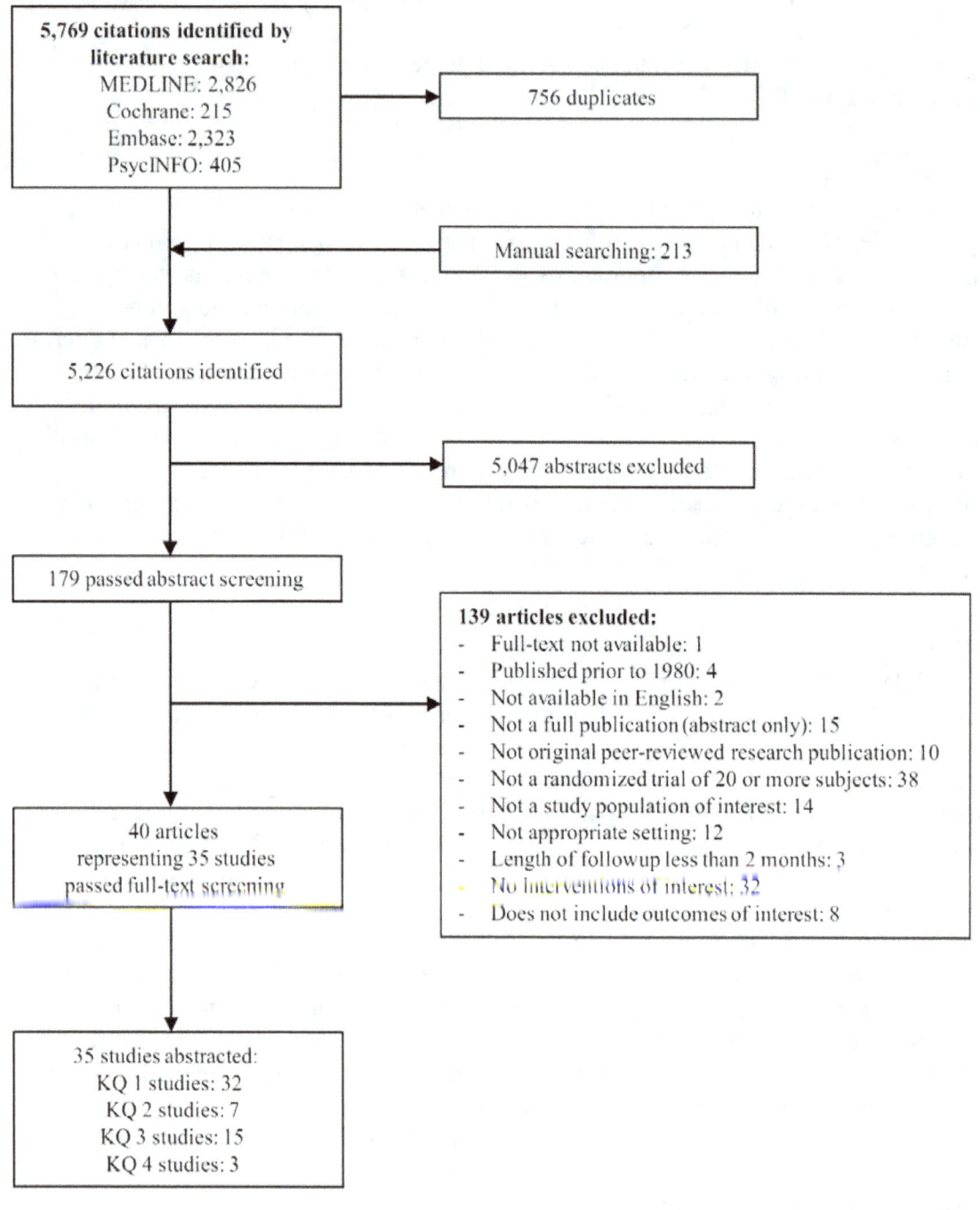

KQ = Key Question

Key Question 1. Effectiveness of Weight-Management Interventions

Key points are:

- Of the 32 studies identified, most were specifically designed to control weight gain for individuals with SMI.
- Behavioral interventions were found in a meta-analysis to have a significant advantage over control conditions. We found moderate strength of evidence (SOE) that behavioral interventions are associated with small decreases in weight (about 3 kg) compared with controls.
- Switching to or adding adjunctive aripiprazole, adding the anticonvulsant medications topiramate and zonisamide, or adding metformin yielded small to moderate weight loss (low SOE).
- There was no advantage in favor of nizatidine compared with placebo for the management of weight gain among patients with SMI (low SOE).
- No studies evaluated the weight loss medication orlistat in this population.
- Few studies reported effects on physical functioning or health-related quality of life, and no studies reported all-cause mortality.

We identified 32 RCTs encompassing 3,473 participants that assessed the effects of weight-management strategies among adults with SMI. Most studies (n=19) were rated fair quality, with 9 studies rated good quality and 4 poor quality. In total, 22 studies targeted weight control, 6 obesity prevention, 3 antipsychotic metabolic effects, and 1 diabetes management. Of the 3,473 participants across the 32 included studies, most were male and white.

We had sufficient studies to perform three meta-analyses: behavioral interventions, the anticonvulsant medications topiramate and zonisamide, and the antihistamine nizatidine compared with placebo control. Other comparisons were synthesized qualitatively. We found moderate SOE that behavioral interventions are associated with small decreases in weight compared with controls (mean difference, -3.13 kg; 95% CI, -4.21 to -2.05). We found low SOE that switching to or adding adjunctive aripiprazole, adding the anticonvulsant medications topiramate and zonisamide (mean difference, -5.11 kg; CI, -9.48 to -0.74), or adding metformin (mean difference, -4.13 kg; 95% CI, -6.58 to -1.68) yield small to moderate weight loss. Nizatidine, an antihistamine, did not show any consistent effect on weight (mean difference, -0.496 kg; CI, -1.256 to 0.266) with a low SOE. The SOE was insufficient for all other interventions. No studies evaluated orlistat, an FDA-approved medication for the treatment of obesity that is also available without prescription at a lower dose.

Key Question 2. Effectiveness of Diabetes-Management Interventions

Key points are:

- Overall, we found insufficient evidence to support any strategy to control glucose. Of the seven studies identified, only one evaluated an intervention specifically designed to target glucose control in individuals with SMI who have diabetes. Two additional studies evaluated interventions targeting nondiabetic individuals who had or were at risk for poor glycemic control. Four studies evaluated interventions targeting weight, with glycemic control as a secondary outcome.
- The interventions represented in these seven studies were ramelteon, antipsychotic switching, metformin, amantadine, and behavioral interventions.

- Just two of the trials found significant advantages for the intervention in controlling HbA1c, with both of these studies involving the use of metformin. Improvements in HbA1c were small.
- Health-related quality of life and serious adverse events were inconsistently reported in the seven trials. Only one study reported effects on physical functioning or health-related quality of life, and no studies reported CVD mortality.

We identified 7 RCTs encompassing 681 participants that assessed the effects of diabetes-management strategies among adults with SMI. Of these studies, one was rated good quality, five fair quality, and one poor quality. Only one study enrolled patients with diabetes and addressed glucose control directly; the other six studies assessed HbA1c as a secondary outcome.

There was an insufficient number of studies to conduct meta-analyses on the effects of any of the intervention classes by HbA1c. Just two of the trials found significant advantages for the intervention in controlling HbA1c, with both of these studies involving the use of metformin, an FDA-approved drug for the treatment of type 2 diabetes.

Key Question 3. Effectiveness of Dyslipidemia-Management Interventions

Key points are:
- Lipid levels have not been a primary target for interventions studied in individuals with SMI. While 15 RCTs reported lipid levels as a secondary outcome (the studies included in this section), no studies evaluated an intervention specifically designed to target lipid levels in individuals with SMI who have or are at risk for dyslipidemia. Hence, the strength of evidence for this KQ 3 is insufficient.
- Interventions known to be effective for managing dyslipidemia, such as medications (e.g., HMG-CoA reductase inhibitors) or dietary interventions, have not been studied in SMI populations. It seems that such interventions should be considered for clinical use, but direct evidence in SMI populations is lacking.
- Behavioral interventions were found in a meta-analysis to have no advantage over usual care for managing low-density lipoprotein (LDL) levels, but this analysis consisted of three small, 3- to 12-month studies aimed primarily at either weight or diabetes management.
- Small improvements in lipids were seen in one study of ramelteon, one study of topiramate, and one study that used a sequenced medication algorithm of amantadine, metformin, and zonisamide.
- Lipid levels improved modestly in two studies of aripiprazole—one that added aripiprazole to chronic clozapine and one that switched patients from olanzapine to aripiprazole. Switching from oral to injectable olanzapine increased LDL cholesterol.

We identified no articles reporting on trials in which the intervention was designed to target lipid levels. Specifically, no study evaluated HMG-CoA reductase inhibitors (statins), niacin, fibrates, or low-fat diets. However, 15 of the eligible studies, involving 2,322 patients, reported on total cholesterol (n=12) or LDL cholesterol (n=14) as a secondary outcome. Most studies (n=8) were rated fair quality, with four studies rated good quality, and three poor quality. The experimental intervention was psychotropic medication in three trials, antipsychotic switching in four trials, behavioral interventions in three trials, neurological agents in three trials, an antihistamine in one trial, and a neurological agent or a biguanide in one trial (this trial was the only one with three arms instead of two). The majority of patients were male, white, and middle-aged.

We had sufficient studies with cohesive intervention strategies to conduct a meta-analysis only for the effect of behavioral interventions on lipid levels. Behavioral interventions focusing on weight loss or diabetes management have no substantial effects on lipids (LDL levels mean difference, 1.91 mg/dl; 95% CI, -6.06 to 9.88). Small benefits were seen when aripiprazole was used as an adjunct or as an antipsychotic-switching strategy, and single studies suggested possible benefit with ramelteon or topiramate. However, SOE was insufficient for all interventions; no strategies were designed to target lipid levels.

Key Question 4. Effectiveness of Multicondition Lifestyle Interventions

Key points are:

- Only three studies evaluated lifestyle interventions. Lifestyle interventions consisted primarily of dietary and exercise components. One study offered additional provisions such as heart rate monitors and financial subsidies to support the exercise component.
- One study reported small to moderate beneficial effects on body mass index (BMI), weight, and cholesterol.
- This good-quality study showed benefit in switching from olanzapine, quetiapine, or risperidone to aripiprazole in the context of a manualized, behaviorally oriented diet and exercise program.
- The effects of the behavioral component of the lifestyle intervention in this study are unknown, since both the intervention and comparison arm received the behavioral component.
- Two studies reported significant benefits of multicondition lifestyle interventions for self-reported health-related quality of life.
- Studies included in KQ 4 varied substantially on methodological rigor and quality variables.
- Overall, the evidence is insufficient to estimate the effects of multicondition lifestyle interventions.

We identified 1 good and 2 fair-quality studies involving 286 patients that assessed the effects of lifestyle interventions on CVD risk factors and related physical health outcomes among adults with SMI. Most participants were male and white. There was an insufficient number of studies with cohesive intervention strategies to conduct a meta-analysis; results are summarized qualitatively. Two studies evaluated multicomponent lifestyle interventions alone, and one evaluated switching from one of three second-generation antipsychotic medications to aripiprazole in combination with a structured diet and exercise program. None of these studies evaluated lifestyle interventions in combination with medications that directly address weight (e.g., orlistat), glucose (e.g., metformin), or lipids (e.g., statins). Studies reported each outcome separately; only one reported an overall CVD risk score, which was unaffected by the intervention. Adding or switching to aripiprazole results in a small benefit on weight (low SOE), but the evidence is insufficient for overall CVD risk. The two multicomponent behavioral interventions did not have a positive effect on the individual CVD risk factors, although one of the two studies showed a large positive effect on health-related quality of life.

Discussion

Key Findings and Strength of Evidence

We identified 35 trials that tested a wide array of pharmacological and behavioral interventions to address one or more CVD risk factors in adults with SMI who have elevated risk for CVD. Given that CVD is the most prevalent cause of death in this population, this is a surprisingly small number of studies. Further, we identified no peer and family support interventions to address elevated CVD risk, nor did we find any interventions designed specifically to address lipids. No interventions targeted individuals with psychotic depression specifically. Outcomes reported were primarily metabolic outcomes such as glucose control or weight; effects on physical function and overall CVD risk (e.g., Framingham Risk Score) were reported infrequently, and all-cause mortality was not reported.

Table A presents a brief overview of key findings by intervention as well as the strength of evidence (SOE) by KQ for major outcomes. The drug classes in our review sometimes included drugs with diverse mechanisms of action. When results varied by drug, we assigned separate SOE. Publication bias was difficult to assess because only a few comparisons had sufficient studies for statistical analysis. For adverse effects, we considered discontinuation due to adverse effects and worsening of psychiatric status as the key outcomes when rating SOE. When the majority of studies reported only one of these outcomes, we considered the evidence for adverse effects incomplete and rated the limited evidence as indirect. In brief, evidence was insufficient for most intervention strategies, and there were too few studies to conduct quantitative synthesis for all outcomes of interest, except for weight.

Table A. Overview of treatment effects and SOE by intervention and major outcomes[a]

Intervention	KQ 1: Weight	KQ 2: Diabetes (HbA1c)	KQ 3: Lipids[b]	Overall CVD Risk and Other Outcomes
Behavioral	Small benefit (-3.1 kg)[a] Moderate SOE[a]	Insufficient SOE	No important effect from weight control interventions Insufficient SOE	1 study assessed health-related quality of life and found no differences Only 2 studies reported discontinuation due to adverse effects Insufficient SOE
Peer or family support	No studies Insufficient SOE	No studies Insufficient SOE	No studies Insufficient SOE	No studies Insufficient SOE
Metformin	Small benefit (-4.1 kg)[a] Low SOE[a]	Insufficient SOE	No studies Insufficient SOE	Insufficient SOE for CVD risk
Topiramate, zonisamide	Small to moderate benefit (-5.1 kg)[a] Low SOE[a]	Insufficient SOE	Possible benefit with topiramate Insufficient SOE	Insufficient SOE for CVD risk
Antihistamine	No benefit[a] Low SOE[a]	Insufficient SOE	Single study did not suggest benefit Insufficient SOE	Insufficient SOE for CVD risk
Other medications	Insufficient SOE	Insufficient SOE	No study suggested possible benefit Insufficient SOE	Insufficient SOE for CVD risk
Antipsychotic switching or adjunctive use	Low SOE for small benefit (-2 to -3 kg) with switching to aripiprazole or adjunctive aripiprazole[a] Insufficient SOE from single studies that found no effect with switching to quetiapine or parenteral olanzapine	Insufficient SOE	Possible benefit with adjunctive or switching to aripiprazole[a] Low SOE[a]	Insufficient SOE for CVD risk Low SOE for possible higher rate of mental health worsening with switching[a]
Multicomponent lifestyle	Insufficient SOE	Insufficient SOE	Insufficient SOE	2 studies suggested benefit for health-related quality of life 1 study reported no benefit on CVD risk score Insufficient SOE

CVD = cardiovascular disease; KQ = Key Question; SOE = strength of evidence
[a]Shaded cells highlight SOE ratings that are above insufficient.
[b]No studies of lipid-focused interventions.

Prior reviews have identified effective treatments for CVD risk factors such as obesity, tobacco use, and hyperlipidemia in *general populations* or in *adults at increased risk for CVD*.[40-42] We specifically excluded from our review evaluations of general health advice, smoking cessation interventions, and models that provide integrated mental health–general medical care because these topics had been the subject of recent high-quality reviews in patients with SMI.[30-34] Tsoi et al.[30,31] found that bupropion more than doubled the rate of smoking abstinence in smokers with schizophrenia without jeopardizing their mental state. There were few studies of other smoking cessation treatments (including nicotine replacement therapy) and no evidence of benefit for these other treatments. In contrast, Tosh et al.[32] found a small number of RCTs evaluating general physical health advice for patients with SMI, and no clear benefit on health outcomes. Bradford et al.[34] found moderately strong evidence that integrated mental health–general medical care improves preventive services, including CVD screening, but limited and inconsistent effects on physical functioning and CVD risk factors.

Our results complement prior reports by examining a broad array of interventions for patients at increased risk for worsening health outcomes due to CVD risk factors such as obesity, hyperlipidemia, diabetes mellitus, or chronic administration of antipsychotic medication that negatively impacts metabolic parameters. Earlier narrative and systematic reviews have focused primarily on behavioral interventions for weight control in patients with schizophrenia or who were on antipsychotic medications.[43-49] These reviews used differing eligibility criteria, with some including observational designs. Despite the differences in methods, the conclusions of these reviews are largely consistent with our findings that behavioral interventions are associated with small improvements in weight. Our review builds on these findings by identifying clear omissions in treatments that are known to be effective in non-SMI populations, including guideline-concordant care, and promising treatment strategies such as aripiprazole, metformin, and topiramate, which deserve further investigation.

Applicability

In our review, only 15 of 35 trials were conducted in the United States, and most studies (n=21) were classified as efficacy studies and were relatively short in duration. Studies typically enrolled midlife adults; none specifically enrolled older adults. Women, as well as racial minorities, were well represented overall but underrepresented for some specific comparisons. Most studies were conducted in mental health outpatient settings, typical of the principal locus of medical care for patients with SMI; none were conducted in patient-centered medical homes or in settings that integrated mental health with general medical services. None were classified as effectiveness studies, but for many interventions, initial studies are justifiably designed to answer the question "Can it work under ideal conditions?" before moving to a test of effectiveness. Probably the most important constraint on applicability is the inconsistent reporting of the CVD-related outcomes of interest and the nearly total lack of reporting (only reported in one study) for overall CVD risk indices (e.g., Framingham Risk Score).

Implications for Clinical and Policy Decisionmaking

The U.S. Preventive Services Task Force makes recommendations for CVD screening in adults, including blood pressure[50] and tobacco use,[51] screening for diabetes in patients with elevated blood pressure,[52] and lipid screening in midlife adults or young adults at increased risk for CVD.[53] Increasing guideline-concordant care for individuals with SMI—given the current lack of evidence for SMI-specific interventions—could be considered a starting point for minimizing CVD risk in patients with SMI. These guidelines for the general population should then be modified to consider the special risks for patients with SMI.

Our review, together with other reviews on interventions to decrease CVD risk in patients with or without SMI, suggests a few actionable strategies and others requiring further study. For weight control, moderate evidence supports behavioral interventions, and more limited evidence supports metformin, topiramate, or aripiprazole as an adjunctive or antipsychotic-switching strategy. All of these interventions yield small to moderate effects, and the benefits must be weighed against the potential harms. Because only limited data on harms were reported in the trials examined, data from non-SMI populations should be incorporated into decisionmaking. Data are much more limited for effects on average glucose control or lipid levels in patients at increased risk. The antihistamine nizatidine was not effective for any CVD risk factor and is unlikely to be a useful treatment. Other reviews identify bupropion as the best-supported treatment for smoking cessation;[30,31] nicotine replacement therapy is effective in non-SMI populations but has not been adequately studied in patients with schizophrenia, bipolar disorder, or psychotic depression. Other reviews identified tailored mood management in patients with depressive symptoms[54,55] and behavioral support interventions in individuals with mental illness as potentially effective.[56] Although the evidence is limited, the meta-finding is that, of the interventions tested in SMI populations to date, effects on intermediate outcomes (e.g., weight) are similar to the effects found in the general population.

Studies of guideline adherence show significant gaps between current practice and recommendations for CVD risk screening and followup.[57] Studies show screening rates ranging from about 10 to 26 percent for lipids and 22 to 52 percent for glucose.[58-61] Data on monitoring of these risk factors in patients treated with second-generation antipsychotics are more limited but also show gaps between guidelines and practice. Assessment and monitoring is only a first step. When abnormalities are detected, they must be addressed, either by the mental health professional or by a general medicine clinician. Integrated mental health–general medical care has shown promise as the optimal way to deliver this care, and the current move to medical homes has the potential to make this type of care more readily available. Unfortunately, few medical home models to date have explicitly included mental health care.[62] Until integrated care is better established and more readily available, there are a number of implementation strategies to consider when a change to a metabolically more neutral antipsychotic is not sufficient to address elevated CVD risk factors. When patients have access to both mental health specialty care and general medical care, it is important that these clinicians coordinate care across issues that may impact both physical and mental health. For example, general medical providers may be aware of the adverse metabolic effects of some psychotropics but are appropriately hesitant to adjust these medications. Coordinating care with the mental health professional about roles and specific strategies for addressing CVD risk factors has the potential to improve care and clinical outcomes.

Research Gaps

We considered PICOTS (population, intervention, comparator, outcomes, timing, and setting) to identify gaps and classifies gaps as due to: (1) insufficient or imprecise information, (2) biased information; (3) inconsistency or unknown consistency, and (4) not the right information.[63] Gaps and recommendations are presented in Table B. Because the list of gaps in evidence is extensive, we suggest general principles for prioritizing research as applied to the population of adults with SMI. Most groups[64] advocate input from multiple stakeholders and consideration of issues such as the burden of disease, the availability of existing treatment options, the likelihood that the new intervention will substantially improve outcomes, practice variation and health disparities, and the feasibility of implementing effective interventions with existing resources. Specific research questions can be evaluated quantitatively, using value-of-information analysis, which employs Bayesian methods to estimate the potential benefits of gathering more information through research.[65] A recent AHRQ white paper used a multiple-stakeholder consensus process to identify patient-centered outcomes research priorities for serious mental illness,[66] and prioritized comparative effectiveness studies of interventions targeting modifiable risk factors such as tobacco abuse, physical exercise, and nutrition.

We also considered the most appropriate research designs for the research gaps. We suggest that observational designs may be particularly appropriate for these applications: (1) evaluating interventions proven effective in non-SMI populations, (2) testing the *effectiveness* of interventions demonstrated efficacious in tightly controlled trials, and (3) formulating hypotheses to be tested in RCTs. RCTs may be particularly useful for interventions specifically tailored for SMI populations and for drugs, or drug strategies (e.g., antipsychotic switching), that are used primarily in this population. Although we recommend multicenter RCTs to address some evidence gaps, we are aware that there are particular challenges to conducting RCTs in this population. For example, individuals with SMI have been routinely excluded from large cardiovascular trials—limiting opportunities to participate in research. Also, behavioral interventions may be affected by limited access to healthy foods or opportunities for exercise because many individuals with SMI are in lower socioeconomic status groups. Some important outcomes, such as cardiovascular events, may take large sample sizes and long followup periods to evaluate.

Table B. Evidence gaps and future research for adults with SMI

PICOTS	Evidence Gap	Reason	Type of Studies To Consider
Patients	Limited data for patients with conditions other than schizophrenia	Insufficient information	Single and multisite RCTs Quasi-experimental or clinical records-based observational studies
	No data in older adults who have more comorbid medical illness	Insufficient information	Single and multisite RCTs Quasi-experimental or clinical records-based observational studies
	Few studies of ethnic and racial minorities	Insufficient information	Single and multisite RCTs Quasi-experimental or clinical records-based observational studies
Interventions	No interventions evaluating peer and family support interventions	Insufficient information	Single and multisite RCTs
	No studies on the effects of the most recently approved second-generation antipsychotics such as paliperidone, iloperidone, asenapine, and lurasidone	Insufficient information	Single and multisite RCTs Quasi-experimental or clinical records-based observational studies
	Limited evidence about the benefits and harms of switching from one antipsychotic to another on metabolic parameters	Insufficient information	Secondary analyses of existing studies such as the CATIE trial or large observational datasets
	No studies comparing optimized antipsychotic management (e.g., start with or switch to drugs with more favorable metabolic profiles) with continuing current antipsychotics in responders and treating adverse metabolic effects directly using treatments (e.g., statins) with known efficacy	Insufficient information	Single and multisite RCTs Quasi-experimental studies
	Few multimodal interventions (e.g., robust behavioral and pharmacological treatments) and few multicondition interventions (interventions that address multiple CVD risk factors)	Insufficient information	Single and multisite RCTs
	Few evaluations of smoking cessation interventions other than bupropion[a]	Insufficient information	Single and multisite RCTs Quasi-experimental or clinical records-based observational studies
	Few studies evaluating integrated mental health and general medical care[a]	Insufficient information	Single and multisite RCTs Quasi-experimental or clinical records-based observational studies
	Uncertainty about the key characteristics of successful behavioral interventions (e.g., tailoring, dose, duration, delivery mode, individual vs. group)	Insufficient information Not the right information	Improved intervention reporting Single and multisite RCTs Systematic reviews
	Uncertainty about the details of the intervention	Not the right information	Manuals provided to promote replication/implementation of successful interventions
	Interventions to improve guideline concordant care	Insufficient information	Single and multisite RCTs Quasi-experimental studies
Comparators	Few studies comparing two active interventions	Insufficient information	Single and multisite RCTs comparing effective treatments Quasi-experimental or clinical records-based observational studies

Table B. Evidence gaps and future research for adults with SMI (continued)

	Evidence Gap	Reason	Type of Studies to Consider
Outcomes	Uncertain effects on overall CVD risk or cardiovascular events	Insufficient information	Risk indices (e.g., Framingham Risk Score) and/or cardiovascular events used as outcome measures
	Intervention adherence	Insufficient information	Improved study reporting
	Uncertainty about adverse effects on mental health status and other serious adverse effects, specifically in individuals with SMI	Insufficient information	Studies that define and report the proportion of patients for whom mental health status worsens Improved reporting of adverse effects
Timing	Few studies with outcomes measured beyond 6 months	Insufficient information	RCTs with longer term followup Quasi-experimental or observational studies
Setting	Lack of studies designed to evaluate "real world" effects of the intervention (effectiveness studies)	Insufficient information	RCTs or quasi-experimental studies with broad inclusion criteria, conducted in community practices, with long-term followup and which include clinically important outcomes such as physical functioning, cardiovascular events, and adverse events Improved reporting of efficacy–effectiveness characteristics

CATIE = Clinical Antipsychotic Trials in Intervention Effectiveness; CVD = cardiovascular disease; PICOTS = patients, interventions, comparators, outcomes, timing, setting; RCT = randomized controlled trial; SMI = serious mental illness.
[a]Research gaps from prior high-quality systematic reviews that were identified during the topic refinement phase of this review and are described briefly in this report.

Conclusions

In summary, individuals with SMI are at risk for increased CVD—in part due to health behaviors, direct effects of the illness, and adverse effects from some treatments. Prior reviews identified bupropion as effective for smoking cessation, and integrated general medical and mental health care as effective for CVD screening. In our review, surprisingly few studies addressed one or more CVD risk factors in patients with SMI, and most studies were skewed toward efficacy trials. Behavioral interventions, switching to or adding adjunctive aripiprazole, adding anticonvulsant medications topiramate and zonisamide, or adding metformin yield small to moderate weight loss compared with controls. We found insufficient evidence to support any strategy to control glucose. We found limited support of behavioral interventions focusing on weight loss or diabetes management or lipid control; SOE was insufficient for all other interventions. We found no studies testing a number of important interventions (e.g., orlistat, statins) known to be effective in non-SMI populations. Comparative effectiveness trials are needed that test multimodal strategies, known effective agents in non-SMI population (e.g., statins), and antipsychotic management strategies. However, in the absence of evidence for SMI-specific interventions, guideline-concordant care for individuals with SMI may help mitigate the unequal burden of CVD that SMI populations sustain.

References

1. National Institute of Mental Health. Statistics. www.nimh.nih.gov/ statistics/index.shtml. Accessed June 22, 2012.

2. National Institute of Mental Health. Statistics. Schizophrenias. www.nimh.nih.gov/statistics/1SCHIZ.shtml. Accessed June 22, 2012.

3. Epstein J., Barker P, Vorburger M, et al. Serious Mental Illness and its Co-occurrence With Substance Use Disorders, 2002 (DHHS Publication No. SMA 04-3905, Analytic Series A-24). Rockville, MD: Substance Abuse and Mental Health Services Administration, Office of Applied Studies. www.samhsa.gov/data/CoD/ CoD.pdf. Accessed June 22, 2012.

4. Chang C-K, Hayes R, Broadbent M, et al. All-cause mortality among people with serious mental illness (SMI), substance use disorders, and depressive disorders in southeast London: a cohort study. BMC Psychiatry. 2010;10(1):77. PMID: 20920287.

5. Brown AS, Birthwhistle J. Excess mortality of mental illness. Br J Psychiatry. 1996;169(3):383-4. PMID: 8879735.

6. Hsu JH, Chien IC, Lin CH, et al. Incidence of diabetes in patients with schizophrenia: a population-based study. Can J Psychiatry. 2011;56(1):19-26. PMID: 21324239.

7. Dixon L, Weiden P, Delahanty J, et al. Prevalence and correlates of diabetes in national schizophrenia samples. Schizophr Bull. 2000;26(4):903-12. PMID: 11087022.

8. van Winkel R, De Hert M, Van Eyck D, et al. Prevalence of diabetes and the metabolic syndrome in a sample of patients with bipolar disorder. Bipolar Disord. 2008;10(2):342-8. PMID: 18271914.

9. Bresee LC, Majumdar SR, Patten SB, et al. Prevalence of cardiovascular risk factors and disease in people with schizophrenia: a population-based study. Schizophr Res. 2010;117(1):75-82. PMID: 20080392.

10. Weiner M, Warren L, Fiedorowicz JG. Cardiovascular morbidity and mortality in bipolar disorder. Ann Clin Psychiatry. 2011;23(1):40-7. PMID: 21318195.

11. Kilbourne AM, Morden NE, Austin K, et al. Excess heart-disease-related mortality in a national study of patients with mental disorders: identifying modifiable risk factors. Gen Hosp Psychiatry. 2009;31(6):555-63. PMID: 19892214.

12. Miller BJ, Paschall CB, 3rd, Svendsen DP. Mortality and medical comorbidity among patients with serious mental illness Psychiatr Serv. 2006;57(10):1482-7. PMID: 17035569.

13. Fagiolini A, Goracci A. The effects of undertreated chronic medical illnesses in patients with severe mental disorders. J Clin Psychiatry. 2009;70 Suppl 3:22-9. PMID: 19570498.

14. Ryan MC, Collins P, Thakore JH. Impaired fasting glucose tolerance in first-episode, drug-naive patients with schizophrenia. Am J Psychiatry. 2003;160(2):284-9. PMID: 12562574.

15. Kupfer DJ. The increasing medical burden in bipolar disorder. JAMA. 2005;293(20):2528-30. PMID: 15914754.

16. McCreadie RG. Diet, smoking and cardiovascular risk in people with schizophrenia: descriptive study. Br J Psychiatry. 2003;183:534-9. PMID: 14645025.

17. McElroy SL. Obesity in patients with severe mental illness: overview and management. J Clin Psychiatry. 2009;70 Suppl 3:12-21. PMID: 19570497.

18. Fountoulakis KN, Siamouli M, Panagiotidis P, et al. Obesity and smoking in patients with schizophrenia and normal controls: a case-control study. Psychiatry Res. 2010;176(1):13-6. PMID: 20079934.

19. Brown S, Birtwistle J, Roe L, et al. The unhealthy lifestyle of people with schizophrenia. Psychol Med. 1999;29(3):697-701. PMID: 10405091.

20. Kilbourne AM, Rofey DL, McCarthy JF, et al. Nutrition and exercise behavior among patients with bipolar disorder. Bipolar Disord. 2007;9(5):443-52. PMID: 17680914.

21. Newcomer JW. Metabolic considerations in the use of antipsychotic medications: a review of recent evidence. J Clin Psychiatry. 2007;68 Suppl 1:20-7. PMID: 17286524.

22. Kendler KS, Gallagher TJ, Abelson JM, et al. Lifetime prevalence, demographic risk factors, and diagnostic validity of nonaffective psychosis as assessed in a US community sample. The National Comorbidity Survey. Arch Gen Psychiatry. 1996;53(11):1022-31. PMID: 8911225.

23. Viron MJ, Stern TA. The impact of serious mental illness on health and healthcare. Psychosomatics. 2010;51(6):458-65. PMID: 21051676.

24. Desai MM, Rosenheck RA, Druss BG, et al. Receipt of nutrition and exercise counseling among medical outpatients with psychiatric and substance use disorders. J Gen Intern Med. 2002;17(7):556-60. PMID: 12133146.

25. Druss BG, Rosenheck RA, Desai MM, et al. Quality of preventive medical care for patients with mental disorders. Med Care. 2002;40(2):129-36. PMID: 11802085.

26. Green JL, Gazmararian JA, Rask KJ, et al. Quality of diabetes care for underserved patients with and without mental illness: site of care matters. Psychiatr Serv. 2010;61(12):1204-10. PMID: 21123404.

27. Frayne SM, Halanych JH, Miller DR, et al. Disparities in diabetes care: impact of mental illness. Arch Intern Med. 2005;165(22):2631-8. PMID: 16344421.

28. Mitchell AJ, Lord O. Do deficits in cardiac care influence high mortality rates in schizophrenia? A systematic review and pooled analysis. J Psychopharmacol. 2010;24(4 Suppl):69-80. PMID: 20923922.

29. Peck MC, Scheffler RM. An analysis of the definitions of mental illness used in state parity laws. Psychiatr Serv. 2002;53(9):1089-95. PMID: 12221306.

30. Tsoi DT, Porwal M, Webster AC. Interventions for smoking cessation and reduction in individuals with schizophrenia. Cochrane Database Syst Rev. 2010(6):CD007253. PMID: 20556777.

31. Tsoi DT, Porwal M, Webster AC. Efficacy and safety of bupropion for smoking cessation and reduction in schizophrenia: systematic review and meta-analysis. Br J Psychiatry. 2010;196(5):346-53. PMID: 20435957.

32. Tosh G, Clifton A, Bachner M. General physical health advice for people with serious mental illness. Cochrane Database Syst Rev. 2011;2:CD008567. PMID: 21328308.

33. Tosh G, Clifton A, Mala S, et al. Physical health care monitoring for people with serious mental illness. Cochrane Database Syst Rev. 2010(3):CD008298. PMID: 20238365.

34. Bradford DW, Slubicki MN, McDuffie JR, et al. Effects of care models to improve general medical outcomes for individuals with serious mental illness. VA-ESP Project #09-010; [In press.].

35. Agency for Healthcare Research and Quality. Methods Guide for Effectiveness and Comparative Effectiveness Reviews. Rockville, MD: Agency for Healthcare Research and Quality. www.effectivehealthcare.ahrq.gov/index.cfm/search-for-guides-reviews-and-reports/?pageaction=displayproduct&productid=318. Accessed June 12, 2012.

36. Evidence-based Practice Center Systematic Review Protocol. Project Title:Strategies to Improve Cardiovascular Risk Factors in People With Serious Mental Illness: A Comparative Effectiveness Review. January 17, 2012. effectivehealthcare.ahrq.gov/index.cfm/search-for-guides-reviews-and-reports/?productid=933&pageaction=displayproduct. Accessed September 24, 2012.

37. Higgins JP, Thompson SG. Quantifying heterogeneity in a meta-analysis. Statistics in Medicine. 2002;21(11):1539-58. PMID: 12111919.

38. Owens DK, Lohr KN, Atkins D, et al. AHRQ series paper 5: Grading the strength of a body of evidence when comparing medical interventions—Agency for Healthcare Research and Quality and the Effective Health-Care Program. J Clin Epidemiol. 2010;63(5):513-23. PMID: 19595577.

39. Atkins D, Chang SM, Gartlehner G, et al. Assessing applicability when comparing medical interventions: AHRQ and the Effective Health-Care Program. J Clin Epidemiol. 2011;64(11):1198-207. PMID: 21463926.

40. Leblanc ES, O'Connor E, Whitlock EP, et al. Effectiveness of primary care relevant treatments for obesity in adults: a systematic evidence review for the U.S. Preventive Services Task Force. Ann Intern Med. 2011;155(7):434-47. PMID: 21969342.

41. Cahill K, Stead LF, Lancaster T. Nicotine receptor partial agonists for smoking cessation. Cochrane Database of Systematic Reviews. 2011 Feb 16;(2):CD006103. PMID: 21328282.

42. Evidence-based Practice Center Systematic Review Protocol. Project Title: Comparative Effectiveness of Approaches to Weight Maintenance in Adults. www.effectivehealthcare.ahrq.gov/index.cfm/search-for-guides-reviews-and-reports/?productid=824&pageaction=displayproduct. Accessed June 22, 2012.

43. Verhaeghe N, De Maeseneer J, Maes L, et al. Effectiveness and cost-effectiveness of lifestyle interventions on physical activity and eating habits in persons with severe mental disorders: A systematic review. Int J Behav Nutr Phys Act. 2011 Apr 11;8:28. PMID: 21481247.

44. Happell B, Davies C, Scott D. Health behaviour interventions to improve physical health in individuals diagnosed with a mental illness: a systematic review. Int J Ment Health Nurs. 2012;21(3):236-47. PMID: 22533331.

45. Cabassa LJ, Ezell JM, Lewis-Fernandez R. Lifestyle interventions for adults with serious mental illness: a systematic literature review. Psychiatr Serv. 2010;61(8):774-82. PMID: 20675835.

46. Bartels S, Desilets R. Health Promotion Programs for People With Serious Mental Illness (Prepared by the Dartmouth Health Promotion Research Team). Washington, D.C. SAMHSA-HRSA Center for Integrated Health Solutions. January 2012. www.integration.samhsa.gov/Health_Promotion_White_Paper_Bartels_Final_Document.pdf. Accessed September 17, 2012.

47. Wildes JE, Marcus MD, Fagiolini A. Obesity in patients with bipolar disorder: a biopsychosocial-behavioral model. J Clin Psychiatry. 2006;67(6):904-15. PMID: 16848650.

48. Loh C, Meyer JM, Leckband SG. A comprehensive review of behavioral interventions for weight management in schizophrenia. Ann Clin Psychiatry. 2006;18(1):23-31. PMID: 16517450.

49. Gabriele JM, Dubbert PM, Reeves RR. Efficacy of behavioural interventions in managing atypical antipsychotic weight gain. Obes Rev. 2009;10(4):442-55. PMID: 19389059.

50. U.S. Preventive Services Task Force. Screening for High Blood Pressure: U.S. Preventive Services Task Force Reaffirmation Recommendation Statement. AHRQ Publication No. 08-05105-EF-2, December 2007. First published in Ann Intern Med 2007:147-783-786. www.uspreventiveservicestaskforce.org/uspstf07/hbp/hbprs.htm. Accessed June 15, 2012.

51. U.S. Preventive Services Task Force. Counseling to Prevent Tobacco Use and Tobacco-Caused Disease Recommendation Statement. www.uspreventiveservicestaskforce.org/3rduspstf/tobacccoun/tobcounrs.htm. Accessed June 15, 2012.

52. Norris SL, Kansagara D, Bougatsos C, et al. Screening for Type 2 Diabetes: Update of 2003 Systematic Evidence Review for the U.S. Preventive Services Task Force. Evidence Synthesis No. 61. AHRQ Publication No. 08-05116-EF-1. Rockville, Maryland: Agency for Healthcare Research and Quality. June 2008. www.ncbi.nlm.nih.gov/books/NBK33981/. Accessed June 15, 2012.

53. Helfand M, Carson S. Screening for Lipid Disorders in Adults: Selective Update of 2001 U.S. Preventive Services Task Force Review. Evidence Synthesis No. 49. Rockville, MD: Agency for Healthcare Research and Quality, April 2008. AHRQ Publication no. 08-05114-EF-1. www.ncbi.nlm.nih.gov/books/NBK33494/. Accessed June 15, 2012.

54. Gierisch JM, Bastian LA, Calhoun PS, et al. Smoking cessation interventions for patients with depression: a systematic review and meta-analysis. J Gen Intern Med. 2012;27(3):351-60. PMID: 22038468.

55. Gierisch JM, Bastian LA, Calhoun PS, et al. Comparative Effectiveness of Smoking Cessation Treatments for Patients With Depression: A Systematic Review and Meta-analysis of the Evidence. VA-ESP Project #09-010; 2010.

56. Bryant J, Bonevski B, Paul C, et al. A systematic review and meta-analysis of the effectiveness of behavioural smoking cessation interventions in selected disadvantaged groups. Addiction. 2011;106(9):1568-85. PMID: 21489007.

57. Mitchell AJ, Delaffon V, Vancampfort D, et al. Guideline concordant monitoring of metabolic risk in people treated with antipsychotic medication: systematic review and meta-analysis of screening practices. Psychol Med. 2012;42(1):125-47. PMID: 21846426.

58. Haupt DW, Rosenblatt LC, Kim E, et al. Prevalence and predictors of lipid and glucose monitoring in commercially insured patients treated with second-generation antipsychotic agents. Am J Psychiatry. 2009;166(3):345-53. PMID: 19147694.

59. Morrato EH, Newcomer JW, Kamat S, et al. Metabolic screening after the American Diabetes Association's consensus statement on antipsychotic drugs and diabetes. Diabetes Care. 2009;32(6):1037-42. PMID: 19244091.

60. Morrato EH, Druss B, Hartung DM, et al. Metabolic testing rates in 3 state Medicaid programs after FDA warnings and ADA/APA recommendations for second-generation antipsychotic drugs. Arch Gen Psychiatry. 2010;67(1):17-24. PMID: 20048219.

61. Morrato EH, Druss BG, Hartung DM, et al. Small area variation and geographic and patient-specific determinants of metabolic testing in antipsychotic users. Pharmacoepidemiol Drug Saf. 2011;20(1):66-75. PMID: 21182154.

62. Williams JW, Jackson GL, Powers BJ, et al. Closing the Quality Gap Series: Revisiting the State of the Science. The Patient-Centered Medical Home. (Prepared by the Duke Evidence-based Practice Center under Contract No. 290-2007-10066-I.) Rockville, MD. Agency for Healthcare Research and Quality. [in press].

63. Robinson KA, Saldanha IJ, Mckoy NA. Frameworks for Determining Research Gaps During Systematic Reviews. Methods Future Research Needs Report No. 2. (Prepared by the Johns Hopkins University Evidence-based Practice Center under Contract No. 290-2007-10061-I.) AHRQ Publication No. 11-EHC043-EF. Rockville, MD: Agency for Healthcare Research and Quality. June 2011. www.effectivehealthcare.ahrq.gov/reports/final.cfm. Accessed May 22, 2012.

64. Patient-Centered Outcomes Research Institute. Draft National Priorities for Research and Research Agenda. Version 1. January 23, 2012. www.pcori.org/assets/PCORI-Draft-National-Priorities-and-Research-Agenda.pdf. Accessed February 4, 2013.

65. Myers E, McBroom AJ, Shen L, et al. Value-of-Information Analysis for Patient-Centered Outcomes Research Prioritization. Report prepared by the Duke Evidence-based Practice Center. Patient-Centered Outcomes Research Institute. March 2012.

66. Jonas D, Mansfield AJ, Curtis P, et al. Identifying Priorities for Patient-Centered Outcomes Research for Serious Mental Illness. Research White Paper. (Prepared by the RTI-UNC Institute Evidence-based Practice Center under Contract No. 290-2007-10056-I.) AHRQ Publication No. 11-EHC066-EF. Rockville, MD: Agency for Healthcare Research and Quality. September 2011. www.effectivehealthcare.ahrq.gov/reports/final.cfm.

Glossary

AHRQ	Agency for Healthcare Research and Quality
CI	confidence interval
CVD	cardiovascular disease
df	degrees of freedom
HR	hazard ratio
HRQOL	health-related quality of life
kg	kilogram
KQ	Key Question
MI	myocardial infarction
NA	not available
NR	not reported
OR	odds ratio
PICOTS	population, intervention, comparator, outcomes, timing, setting
QOL	quality of life
RCT	randomized controlled trial
ROB	risk of bias
RR	risk ratio
SMI	serious mental illness
SOE	strength of evidence
TEP	Technical Expert Panel

Introduction

Background

Serious Mental Illness and Cardiovascular Health

Serious mental illness (SMI) is defined generally as a major mental or behavioral disorder, causing substantial impairment in multiple areas of daily functioning. SMI includes disorders such as schizophrenia and bipolar disorder, but not isolated substance abuse or developmental disorders. SMI affects about 4 to 8 percent of adults.[1-3] Individuals with SMI have shortened life expectancies relative to the general population to an extent that is not explained by suicide and accidents alone.[4,5] This population experiences higher rates of morbidity from multiple general medical conditions, including diabetes[6-8] and cardiovascular disease (CVD).[9-11] Among patients using the public mental health system, heart disease was the leading cause of death.[12] This excess of CVD-related mortality may be due to a number of factors including direct effects of the illness, medications used to treat SMI, modifiable behavioral risk factors, and disparities in access and quality of health care.

For CVD, mental illness may be an independent risk factor that acts both directly through physiological effects such as underlying genetic vulnerabilities, or indirectly through effects on an individual's access to or interaction with the health care system.[13-15] Modifiable CVD risk factors, such as smoking,[16] obesity,[17,18] and physical inactivity[19,20] are highly prevalent among adults with SMI. Adverse effects of psychotropic drugs (notably second-generation antipsychotics) also may contribute to the development of CVD by increasing the risk of conditions such as hyperglycemia, hyperlipidemia, and obesity.[21] Lower socioeconomic status is more common in individuals with SMI[22,23] and may limit access to healthy food, opportunities for physical exercise (e.g., walkable neighborhoods and access to fitness facilities), and high-quality medical care. Numerous studies have demonstrated disparities in the quality of general medical care provided to individuals with SMI.[24-28] Given these issues, identifying intervention strategies that address CVD risk in individuals with SMI is a pressing priority to avoid early morbidity and mortality.

Context of Care for Adults With SMI

In contrast to individuals with less severe mental disorders, who largely receive mental health treatment in primary care settings, most individuals with SMI receive mental health treatment in specialized mental health settings. The normative treatment setting for individuals with SMI is outpatient treatment, with acute inpatient treatment for severe exacerbations. A minority of individuals with severe and treatment-resistant symptoms receive long-term inpatient treatment. Furthermore, general medical services have less commonly been offered in sites colocated in mental health settings[29,30] or by those who are dually trained in both a mental health and a general medical discipline.[31] Consequently, people with SMI receive fewer preventive medical services[24,25] and less frequent guideline-concordant treatment to manage chronic physical illnesses such as diabetes[26,27] and CVD.[28] In addition to reduced quality of care for general medical services, multiple studies have demonstrated reduced access to outpatient general medical care among individuals with SMI. The results of an analysis of a nationally representative survey[32] showed that individuals with psychotic disorders and bipolar disorder, but not major depression, were less likely than the general population to have a primary care provider even after controlling for demographics, income, and insurance status.

Current Treatment Approaches

Managing CVD risk in individuals with SMI includes standard pharmacological and behavioral interventions used in the general population (Table 1) as well as treatments specific to this population (e.g., antipsychotic medication–switching to manage adverse effects). Multicondition lifestyle interventions such as combinations of physical activity promotion and nutrition counseling with medical management of chronic medical conditions (e.g., hyperlipidemia) may be used to manage CVD risk factors in individuals with SMI. In addition, peer support interventions have been used to improve mental health outcomes and show promise in improving general medical outcomes;[33] family interventions may have this potential as well. However, interventions and treatments used to improve CVD risk may vary importantly in efficacy, adverse effects, complexity of regimen, need for monitoring, costs, and potential for drug-drug and drug-disease interactions.

The *efficacy* of most pharmacological agents used to reduce CVD risk is expected to be similar in patients with SMI when compared with general populations, but the potential for more severe or higher frequency adverse effects may be greater in individuals with SMI than in general populations due to drug-drug interactions (e.g., thiazides and lithium) or drug-disease interactions (e.g., varenicline and mood disorders). For behavioral interventions, direct effects of SMI and the limited social and economic support systems often available to these individuals may decrease *effectiveness*. To be optimally effective, health behavior interventions used in the general population to manage CVD risk may benefit from customization to the context and needs of individuals with SMI. Given the broad range of potential interventions and uncertainty about the effectiveness of competing strategies, an evidence synthesis was requested to inform guidelines and policy decisions.

Table 1. Selected pharmacological treatments and behavioral strategies to manage CVD risk factors

Comorbid Risk Factors in Adults With SMI	Pharmacological Treatments	Behavioral Strategies
Obesity	Orlistat Metformin Amantadine Topiramate Diethylpropion Phentermine Antipsychotic medication–switching	Patient education Behavioral counseling Exercise interventions Nutrition interventions Weight loss program Patient-focused strategies to optimize adherence Peer and family support interventions
Hyperglycemia/diabetes mellitus	Standard pharmacological treatment (multiple agents) Antipsychotic medication–switching	Patient education Patient-focused strategies to optimize adherence Behavioral counseling Exercise interventions Nutrition interventions Weight loss program Peer and family support interventions
Hyperlipidemia	Statins, fibrates, niacin, etc. (standard treatment) Antipsychotic medication–switching	Patient education Exercise program Nutrition counseling Patient-focused strategies to optimize adherence Peer and family support interventions
Hypertension	Standard pharmacologic treatment (multiple agents) Antipsychotic medication–switching	Patient education Patient-focused strategies to optimize adherence Behavioral counseling Relaxation training Exercise interventions Nutrition interventions Weight loss program Peer and family support interventions

SMI = serious mental illness

Scope and Key Questions

Scope of the Review

This comparative effectiveness review was funded by the Agency for Healthcare Research and Quality (AHRQ). The review was designed to evaluate strategies to improve CVD risk factors in adults with SMI. SMI has been defined variously by different groups over time.[34] For the purposes of this evidence review, people with SMI are defined as individuals who have (1) schizophrenia or schizoaffective disorder (or other related primary psychotic disorder), (2) bipolar disorder, or (3) current major depression with psychotic features. We also included studies that enrolled adults with SMI or severe and persistent mental illness (SPMI) but did not specify diagnoses. Individuals with a primary diagnosis of substance abuse, dementia, personality disorder, or mental retardation are excluded from this definition.

To prioritize interventions for review, we examined published systematic reviews of strategies to improve CVD risk factors in individuals with SMI and consulted with our Key Informants. Because we identified recent high-quality reviews of general health advice, interventions for smoking cessation, and models to provide integrated mental health–general medical care, we elected not to cover these interventions again in our review.[35-39] We included randomized controlled trials (RCTs) of the pharmacological and patient-focused behavioral strategies listed in Table 1, along with peer and family support interventions. For patient-level intervention strategies, RCTs yield the highest quality evidence. We included both active and control comparators. Major outcomes of interest for this report are primary CVD risk factors (excluding tobacco use as explained above), physical functioning or health-related quality of life, adverse effects, and all-cause mortality.

Key Questions

With input from our Technical Expert Panel, we constructed Key Questions (KQs) using the general approach of specifying the population of interest, interventions, comparators, outcomes, timing of outcomes, and settings (PICOTS; see the section on "Inclusion and Exclusion Criteria" in the Methods section for details). The draft KQs developed during this process were available for public comment from 28 October 2011 to 28 November 2011. Comments received led to revisions including the addition of a separate KQ for dyslipidemia and the inclusion of peer and family support interventions in the strategies examined for each KQ. The final KQs considered in this comparative effectiveness review were:

KQ 1: What is the effectiveness of weight-management behavioral interventions (e.g., behavioral counseling, health education), peer or family support interventions, pharmacological treatments (e.g., orlistat, topiramate), antipsychotic medication–switching to an antipsychotic with a low or neutral impact on weight, or their combination on weight control and related physical health outcomes (e.g., health-related quality of life, mortality) compared with each other or with usual care (or other control) among adults with serious mental illness (SMI) who are overweight, obese, or taking antipsychotics?

KQ 2: What is the effectiveness of diabetes-management behavioral interventions (e.g., behavioral counseling, health education), peer or family support interventions, pharmacological treatments (e.g., rosiglitazone, metformin), antipsychotic medication–switching to an antipsychotic with a low or neutral impact on glucose level, or their combination on glucose-level control and related physical health outcomes (e.g., health-related quality of life, mortality) compared with each other or with usual care (or other control) among adults with SMI who have diabetes or are taking antipsychotics?

KQ 3: What is the effectiveness of dyslipidemia-management behavioral interventions (e.g., behavioral counseling, health education), peer or family support interventions, pharmacological treatments (e.g., statins), antipsychotic medication–switching to an antipsychotic with a low or neutral impact on lipid levels, or their combination on lipid-level control and related physical health outcomes (e.g., health-related quality of life, mortality) compared with each other or with usual care (or other control) among adults with SMI who have dyslipidemia or are taking antipsychotics?

KQ 4: What is the effectiveness of multicondition lifestyle interventions (e.g., combinations of smoking cessation, physical activity, and nutrition counseling with or without medication management) on cardiovascular risk factors and related physical health outcomes (e.g., health-related quality of life, mortality) among adults with SMI who have cardiovascular disease, elevated cardiovascular risk (e.g., hypertension), or are taking antipsychotics?

Analytic Framework

Figure 1 shows the analytic framework for this systematic review.

The population evaluated in this comparative effectiveness review is adults with SMI who also have at least one of the following conditions: are overweight or obese; have diabetes, dyslipidemia, or CVD; are at elevated CVD risk, or are taking antipsychotic medication and so are at elevated risk for obesity, diabetes, dyslipidemia, or CVD. Intervention strategies considered by the four KQs are (1) behavioral strategies, (2) peer and family support interventions, (3) pharmacological treatments, (4) combinations of behavioral and pharmacological interventions, (5) antipsychotic medication switching, and (6) multicondition lifestyle interventions. The intermediate outcomes considered are weight control, glucose levels, lipid levels, and CVD risk. The final outcomes considered are mortality, physical function, and health-related quality of life. All four KQs consider the adverse effects of treatment interventions.

Organization of This Report

The remainder of this report is organized to describe detailed methods, overview of included studies, and results by KQ. Each Results section describes primary outcomes relevant to the KQ and cross-references other sections for related outcomes. For example, studies evaluating weight loss interventions are summarized in KQ 1 (weight-management behavioral interventions), but secondary outcomes such as effects on glucose and lipid parameters are cross-referenced to the specific KQ that evaluated those interventions. In the Discussion chapter, we present a table summarizing the strength of evidence across outcomes for each type of intervention.

Figure 1. Analytic framework

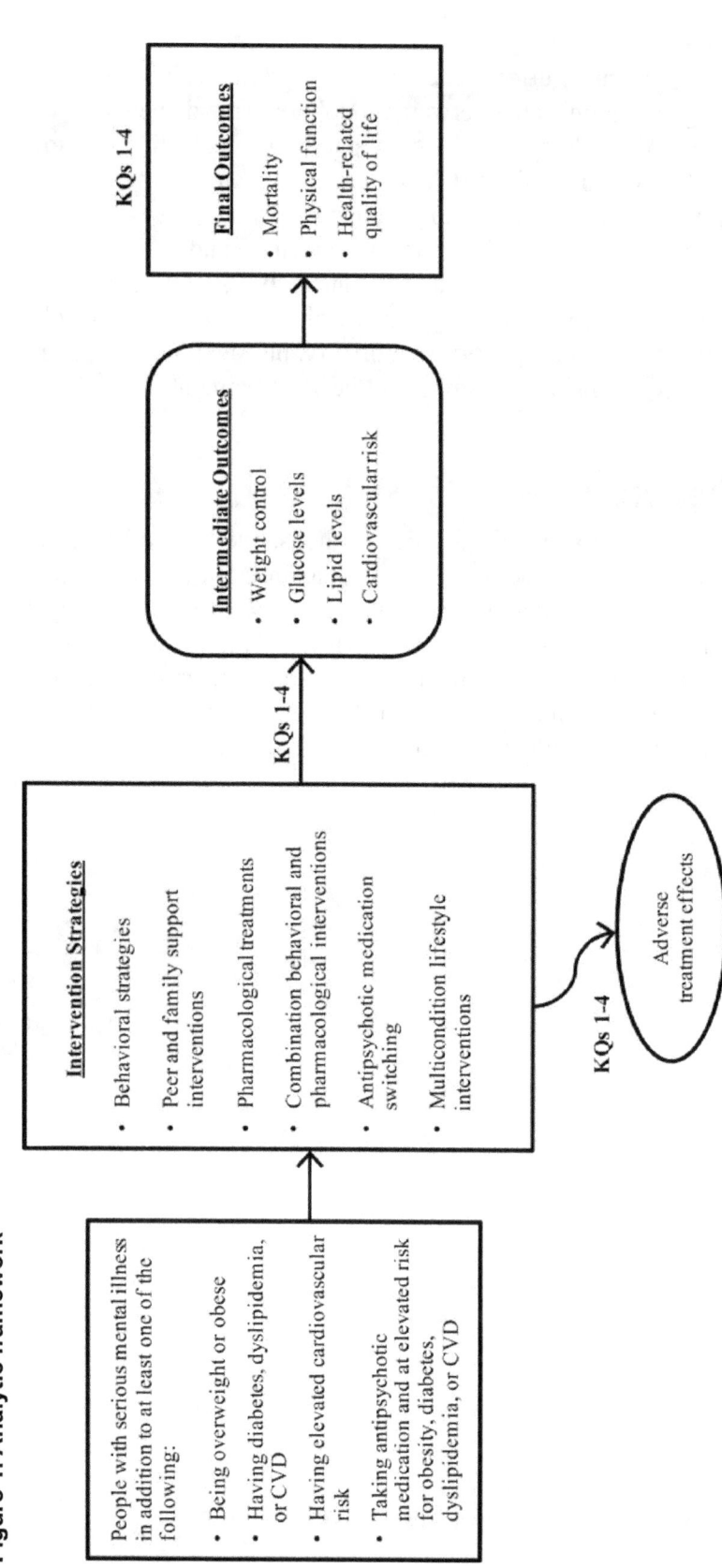

Intervention Strategies

People with serious mental illness in addition to at least one of the following:

- Being overweight or obese
- Having diabetes, dyslipidemia, or CVD
- Having elevated cardiovascular risk
- Taking antipsychotic medication and at elevated risk for obesity, diabetes, dyslipidemia, or CVD

Intervention Strategies

- Behavioral strategies
- Peer and family support interventions
- Pharmacological treatments
- Combination behavioral and pharmacological interventions
- Antipsychotic medication switching
- Multicondition lifestyle interventions

KQs 1-4

Adverse treatment effects

KQs 1-4

Intermediate Outcomes

- Weight control
- Glucose levels
- Lipid levels
- Cardiovascular risk

KQs 1-4

Final Outcomes

- Mortality
- Physical function
- Health-related quality of life

CVD = cardiovascular disease; KQ = Key Question

6

Methods

The methods for this comparative effectiveness review follow those suggested in the AHRQ "Methods Guide for Effectiveness and Comparative Effectiveness Reviews" (available at www.effectivehealthcare.ahrq.gov/methodsguide.cfm; hereafter referred to as the Methods Guide).[40] The main sections in this chapter reflect the elements of the protocol established for the systematic review; certain methods map to the PRISMA checklist.[41]

Topic Refinement and Review Protocol

During the topic refinement stage, we solicited input from Key Informants representing clinicians (psychiatry, psychology, mental health education and treatment), patient advocates, scientific experts, and payers to help define the Key Questions (KQs). The KQs were then posted for a 4-week public comment period, and the comments received were considered in the development of the research protocol. We next convened a TEP comprising clinical, content, and methodological experts to provide input in defining populations, interventions, comparisons, and outcomes, as well as identifying particular studies or databases to search. The Key Informants and members of the TEP were required to disclose any financial conflicts of interest greater than $10,000 and any other relevant business or professional conflicts of interest. Any potential conflicts of interest were balanced or mitigated. Key Informants and members of the TEP did not perform analysis of any kind or contribute to the writing of the report. Members of the TEP were invited to provide feedback on an initial draft of the review protocol which was then refined based on their input, reviewed by AHRQ, and posted for public access at the AHRQ Effective Health Care Web site.[42]

Literature Search Strategy

Sources Searched

To identify the relevant published literature, we searched MEDLINE®, Embase®, PsycINFO®, and the Cochrane Database of Systematic Reviews. Where possible, we used existing validated search filters (such as the Clinical Queries Filters in PubMed®). An experienced search librarian guided all searches. Exact search strings and dates are included in Appendix A. We supplemented the electronic searches with a manual search of citations from a set of key primary and review articles.[43-82] The reference lists for these articles were manually reviewed and cross-referenced against our library of search results, and additional potentially relevant citations were retrieved for screening. All citations were imported into an electronic database (EndNote® X4; Thomson Reuters, Philadelphia, PA).

We used two approaches to identify relevant gray literature: (1) a request for scientific information packets submitted to drug manufacturers and (2) a search of trial records listed in ClinicalTrials.gov (see Appendix A for search date and exact search terms). The search of ClinicalTrials.gov was also used as a mechanism to ascertain publication bias by identifying completed but unpublished studies. During peer and public review of the draft report, we updated the database searches and included any eligible studies identified either through that search or through suggestions from peer and public reviewers.

Inclusion and Exclusion Criteria

The PICOTS criteria used to screen articles for inclusion/exclusion at both the title-and-abstract and full-text screening stages are detailed in Table 2. Given the large number of interventions considered, the higher risk of bias, and complexity of identifying relevant observational studies, we restricted our review to randomized controlled trials.

Table 2. Inclusion and exclusion criteria

Study Characteristic	Inclusion Criteria	Exclusion Criteria
Population	KQs 1–4: According to standardized diagnostic criteria (e.g., DSM-IV, ICD), people ≥18 years of age who currently have (or at any time during the past year had) one of the following: • Schizophrenia or schizoaffective disorder (or other related primary psychotic disorder) • Bipolar disorder • Psychotic depression • No specified diagnosis but are classified as having SMI or severe and persistent mental illness (refer to definition in Introduction of this report). If the sample includes a mixed population of people with SMI, 70% of the sample must comprise the first two conditions above, or the outcomes must be reported separately for this subgroup.	KQs 1–4: • People <18 years of age • People with a primary diagnosis of substance abuse, dementia, personality disorder, or mental retardation. (Studies of individuals with dual diagnoses [e.g., bipolar disorder and substance abuse] are eligible.) • People with a primary diagnosis of other mood disorders
	In addition to these population criteria: KQ 1: • Individuals who are overweight or obese *or* • Individuals who are taking antipsychotics and consequently at increased risk for obesity KQ 2: • Individuals who have diabetes *or* • Individuals who are taking antipsychotics and consequently at risk for elevated glucose levels KQ 3: • Individuals who have dyslipidemia *or* • Individuals who are taking antipsychotics and consequently at risk for elevated lipid levels KQ 4: • Individuals who have cardiovascular disease (CVD) or elevated CVD risk (e.g., hyperlipidemia, hypertension, metabolic syndrome) *or* • Individuals who are taking antipsychotics and consequently at increased risk for CVD	

Table 2. Inclusion and exclusion criteria (continued)

Study Characteristic	Inclusion Criteria	Exclusion Criteria
Interventions[a]	KQs 1–4: • Patient-focused behavioral interventions (e.g., behavioral counseling, patient education, adherence-enhancing interventions), peer or family support interventions, pharmacological treatments, or their combination targeting weight control, glucose levels, or CVD risk profile • Changing from one antipsychotic to another (antipsychotic switching) to manage weight issues *or* elevated glucose levels or CVD risk KQ 4: Multicondition lifestyle interventions (e.g., combinations of behavioral and medication management, broadly conceived behavioral interventions) for more than one CVD risk factor or health condition	KQs 1–4: • Studies evaluating interventions designed to improve psychiatric outcomes • Mass media strategies • Studies of pharmacological agents that are not currently on the U.S. market
Comparators	KQs 1–4: (control conditions) • Usual care • Placebo • Other control (e.g., attention control; waitlist) KQs 1–4: (active comparators) • Patient-focused behavioral interventions, pharmacological treatments, or their combination targeting weight control, glucose levels, or CVD risk profile • Changing from one antipsychotic to another (antipsychotic switching) to manage weight issues, or elevated glucose levels or CVD risk KQ 4: (active comparator) Other multicondition lifestyle interventions	None
Outcomes	KQ 1: Weight control (i.e., weight loss or maintenance of current weight) KQ 2: Glucose level (e.g., hemoglobin A_{1c}) KQ 3: Lipid level (e.g., change in low-density lipoprotein) KQ 4: CVD risk profile (i.e., Framingham CVD scores) or multiple individual components of modifiable CVD risk (e.g., lipid values, blood pressure, smoking status, glucose level) KQs 1–4: • Health-related quality of life • All-cause mortality • Physical function • Serious adverse effects • Adverse effects (i.e., significant worsening of psychiatric status, discontinuations due to serious or nonserious adverse effects)	Article reports only physical function/health-related quality of life outcomes and does not also include a primary CVD risk measure of interest (e.g., weight, glucose level)

Table 2. Inclusion and exclusion criteria (continued)

Study Characteristic	Inclusion Criteria	Exclusion Criteria
Timing	≥2 months	<2 months
Setting	• Outpatient mental health and outpatient general medical settings • Community settings	Intervention delivered primarily in hospital inpatient setting
Study design	RCTs	• Not a clinical study (e.g., editorial, nonsystematic review, letter to the editor, case series) • Prospective and retrospective observational studies • N ≤20
Publications	• English-language only • Peer-reviewed articles • Relevant systematic review, meta-analysis, or methods article (used for background only) • 1980 forward[b]	Non–English-language articles[c]

CVD = cardiovascular disease; DSM-IV, ICD = Diagnostic and Statistical Manual of Mental Disorders, International Classification of Diseases; KQ = Key Question; RCTs = randomized controlled trials; SMI = serious mental illness
[a]Studies were classified by primary study goal (i.e., weight management, diabetes management, CVD management). To meet criteria for inclusion in KQ 4, a study must recruit participants with multiple elevated CVD risk factors and state a goal to improve more than one condition related to CVD risk.
[b]1980 was selected as a date restriction since this was the year the *DSM-III* was introduced.
[c]Given the high volume of English-language publications (including the majority of known important studies), and concerns about the applicability of non-English publication studies to settings in the United States, non–English-language articles were excluded.

Study Selection

Using the prespecified inclusion and exclusion criteria described in Table 2, two investigators independently reviewed titles and abstracts for potential relevance to the KQs. Articles included by either reviewer underwent full-text screening. At the full-text screening stage, two investigators independently reviewed each article to determine if it met eligibility criteria, and indicated a decision to "include" or "exclude" the article for data abstraction. When the paired reviewers arrived at different decisions about whether to include or exclude an article, or about the reason for exclusion, they reconciled the difference through review and discussion, or through a third-party arbitrator if needed. Articles meeting our eligibility criteria were included for data abstraction. Relevant review articles and meta-analyses were flagged for manual searching of references and cross-referencing against the library of citations identified through electronic database searching.

For citations retrieved by searching the gray literature, the above-described procedures were modified such that a single screener initially reviewed all search results; final eligibility of citations for data abstraction was determined by duplicate screening review. All screening decisions were made and tracked in a DistillerSR database (Evidence Partners Inc, Manotick, ON, Canada).

Data Extraction

The investigative team created data abstraction forms and evidence table templates for abstracting data for the KQs. Based on clinical and methodological expertise, a pair of investigators was assigned to abstract data from each eligible article. One investigator abstracted the data, and the second reviewed the article and the accompanying completed abstraction form to check for accuracy and completeness. Quality ratings and efficacy–effectiveness ratings (see below) were completed independently by two investigators. Disagreements were resolved by consensus, or by obtaining a third reviewer's opinion if consensus could not be reached. To aid in both reproducibility and standardization of data collection, researchers received data abstraction instructions directly on each form created specifically for this project within the DistillerSR database.

We designed the data abstraction forms for this project to collect the data required to evaluate the specified eligibility criteria for inclusion in this review, as well as demographic and other data needed for determining outcomes. We gave particular attention to describing the details of the interventions (e.g., pharmacotherapy used, intensity of behavioral interventions), patient characteristics (e.g., SMI diagnosis), and comparators that may be related to outcomes. Data necessary for assessing quality and applicability, as described in the Methods Guide,[40] were also abstracted. When critical data were missing, we contacted study authors. Of the seven authors contacted, five replied with the requested information.

We adapted a previously published efficacy–effectiveness instrument (Appendix B) to assess eight dimensions:[83] (1) setting/practitioner expertise, (2) restrictiveness of eligibility criteria, (3) health outcomes, (4) flexibility of the intervention and study duration, (5) assessment of adverse events, (6) adequate sample size for important health outcomes, (7) intention-to-treat approach to analyses, and (8) identity of the comparison intervention. We developed definitions for each dimension that were specific to the literature reviewed. We rated each of the eight dimensions as effectiveness (score=1) or efficacy (score=0); scores on each dimension were summed and could range from 0–8. Studies were categorized as efficacy (0–2), mixed efficacy–effectiveness (3–5) or effectiveness (6–8) based on summed scores. Simple agreement between investigator pairs was 78 percent and unweighted kappa 0.57, indicating moderate agreement beyond chance for efficacy–effectiveness categories.

Before they were used, abstraction form templates were pilot-tested with a sample of included articles to ensure that all relevant data elements were captured and that there was consistency/reproducibility between abstractors. Forms were revised as necessary before full abstraction of all included articles. Some outcomes were reported only in figures. In these instances, we used the web-based software, EnGauge Digitizer (digitizer.sourceforge.net/) to convert graphical displays to numerical data. Appendix C lists the elements included in the data abstraction forms.

Quality Assessment of Individual Studies

We evaluated the quality of individual studies using the key criteria for RCTs described in the Methods Guide.[40] Criteria of interest included methods of randomization and allocation concealment, similarity of groups at baseline, extent to which outcomes were described, blinding of subjects and providers, blinded assessment of the outcome(s), intention-to-treat analysis, differential loss to followup between the compared groups or overall high loss to followup, and conflicts of interest.

To indicate the summary judgment of the quality of the individual studies, we used the summary ratings of good, fair, or poor based on their adherence to well-accepted standard methodologies and adequate reporting (Table 3). For each study, two investigators independently assigned a summary quality rating; disagreements were resolved by consensus or by discussion with a third investigator if agreement could not be reached. Quality ratings were assigned separately for "hard" outcomes (e.g., mortality, laboratory measurements) and all other outcomes (e.g., health-related quality of life); thus, a given study may have been categorized differently for two individual outcomes reported within that study.

Table 3. Definitions of overall quality ratings

Quality Rating	Description
Good	A study with the least bias; results are considered valid. A good study has a clear description of the population, setting, interventions, and comparison groups; uses a valid approach to allocate patients to alternative treatments; has a low dropout rate; and uses appropriate means to prevent bias, measure outcomes, and analyze and report results.
Fair	A study that is susceptible to some bias but probably not enough to invalidate the results. The study may be missing information, making it difficult to assess limitations and potential problems. As the fair-quality category is broad, studies with this rating vary in their strengths and weaknesses. The results of some fair-quality studies are possibly not valid, while others are probably valid.
Poor	A study with significant bias that may invalidate the results. These studies have serious errors in design, analysis, or reporting; have large amounts of missing information; or have discrepancies in reporting. The results of a poor-quality study are at least as likely to reflect flaws in the study design as to indicate true differences between the compared interventions.

Data Synthesis

We began by summarizing key features of the included studies for each KQ. To the degree that data were available, we abstracted information on study design; patient characteristics; clinical settings; interventions; and intermediate, final, and adverse effects outcomes. We then determined the feasibility of completing a quantitative synthesis (i.e., meta-analysis). Feasibility depended on the volume of relevant literature (≥ 3 studies), conceptual homogeneity of the studies, and completeness of the reporting of results. When a meta-analysis was appropriate, we used random-effects models to quantitatively synthesize the available evidence. For other outcomes we analyzed the results qualitatively. The outcomes amenable to meta-analysis were continuous; we therefore summarized these outcomes by a weighted difference of the means when the same scale (e.g., weight) was used and a standardized mean difference when the scales (e.g., health-related quality of life) differed across studies. We standardized results presentation such that a negative value indicates a greater intervention effect. When needed, we converted reported outcomes to a common unit (e.g., cholesterol from mmol/L to mg/dl). We present summary estimates, standard errors, and confidence intervals in our data synthesis.

We organized our analyses by KQ. When a single study reported outcomes relevant to multiple KQs, it was included in the analyses for each question. For example, a study evaluating a weight-loss intervention that specified weight as the primary outcome—but which also reported effects on glucose and lipid parameters—was described in each relevant KQ. When a study was designed to intervene on more than one CVD risk factor (e.g., metabolic syndrome), it was summarized in KQ 4. We specified, a priori, weight control as measured by change in kilograms (or pounds); hemoglobin A1c (HbA1c) as the preferred measure of glucose control since it reflects average glucose values over a 3-month interval; and total and LDL cholesterol as measures of lipid control. For adverse effects, we report significant worsening of psychiatric status and discontinuations due to adverse effects. Interventions were categorized as behavioral, pharmacological, peer or family support, or multicondition (e.g., specifically targeting more than one condition such as smoking cessation and weight loss). Drug classes were psychotropics, neurologics, metformin, antihistamines, nutritionals (i.e., carnitine), and switching between antipsychotic medications.

We tested for heterogeneity using graphical displays and test statistics (Q statistic), while recognizing that the ability of statistical methods to detect heterogeneity may be limited.[84] The I^2 describes the percentage of total variation across studies due to heterogeneity rather than to chance. Heterogeneity was categorized as low, moderate, or high based on I^2 values of 25 percent, 50 percent, and 75 percent respectively.[84] When there were sufficient studies, we explored heterogeneity in study effects by using subgroup analyses. When there were sufficient studies (n ≥10), we assessed for publication bias using funnel plots and test statistics.[85] All analyses were conducted using Comprehensive Meta-Analysis software (Version 2; Biostat, Englewood, NJ).

Strength of the Body of Evidence

The strength of evidence for each KQ and outcome was assessed using the approach described in the Methods Guide.[40,86] In brief, the approach requires assessment of four domains: risk of bias, consistency, directness, and precision (Table 4).

Table 4. Strength of evidence required domains

Domain	Rating	How Assessed
Quality (risk of bias)	Good Fair Poor	Assessed primarily through study design (RCT vs. observational study) and aggregate study quality
Consistency	Consistent Inconsistent Unknown/not applicable	Assessed primarily through whether effect sizes are generally on the same side of "no effect," the overall range of effect sizes, and statistical measures of heterogeneity
Directness	Direct Indirect	Assessed by whether the evidence involves direct comparisons or indirect comparisons through use of surrogate outcomes or use of separate bodies of evidence
Precision	Precise Imprecise	Based primarily on the size of the confidence intervals of effect estimates, the optimal information size and considerations of whether the confidence interval crossed the clinical decision threshold for using a therapy

RCT = randomized controlled trial

Additional domains were used when appropriate: coherence, and publication bias. These domains were considered qualitatively, and a summary rating of high, moderate, or low strength of evidence was assigned after discussion by two reviewers. In some cases, high, moderate, or low ratings were impossible or imprudent to make; for example, when no evidence was available or when evidence on the outcome was too weak, sparse, or inconsistent to permit any conclusion to be drawn. In these situations, a grade of insufficient was assigned. This four-level rating scale consists of the following definitions:

- High—High confidence that the evidence reflects the true effect. Further research is very unlikely to change our confidence in the estimate of effect.
- Moderate—Moderate confidence that the evidence reflects the true effect. Further research may change our confidence in the estimate of effect and may change the estimate.

- Low—Low confidence that the evidence reflects the true effect. Further research is likely to change the confidence in the estimate of effect and is likely to change the estimate.
- Insufficient—Evidence either is unavailable or does not permit estimation of an effect.

Applicability

We assessed applicability across our KQs using the method described in the Methods Guide.[40,87] In brief, this method uses the PICOTS format as a way to organize information relevant to applicability. The most important issue with respect to applicability is whether the outcomes are different across studies that recruit different populations (e.g., age groups, exclusions for comorbidities) or use different methods to implement the interventions of interest; that is, important characteristics are those that affect baseline (control-group) rates of events, intervention-group rates of events, or both. We used a checklist to guide the assessment of applicability (Appendix C). We used these data to evaluate the applicability to clinical practice, paying special attention to study eligibility criteria, demographic features of the enrolled population in comparison with the target population, characteristics of the intervention used in comparison with care models currently in use, and clinical relevance and timing of the outcome measures. We summarized issues of applicability qualitatively.

Peer Review and Public Commentary

The peer review process is our principal external quality-monitoring device. Nominations for peer reviewers were solicited from several sources, including the TEP and interested Federal agencies. Experts in psychiatry, mental illness, chronic medical conditions, systematic review methodology, pharmacoepidemiology of SMI, public health, and integration of mental health and primary care, along with individuals representing stakeholder and user communities, were invited to provide external peer review of this draft report; AHRQ and an associate editor also provided comments. The draft report was posted on AHRQ's Web site for public comment for 4 weeks, from July 19, 2012, to August 17, 2012. We have addressed reviewer comments, revising the report as appropriate, and have documented our responses in a disposition of comments report available on the AHRQ Web site. A list of peer reviewers is given in the preface of this report.

Results

Introduction

In what follows, we begin by presenting the results of our literature searches. We then provide a brief description of the included studies. The remainder of the chapter is organized by Key Question (KQ). Under each KQ, we begin by listing the key points of the findings, followed by a brief description of included studies, followed by a more detailed synthesis of the evidence. The detailed syntheses are organized by intervention and primary outcomes: cardiovascular risk factor, functional status or health-related quality of life, adverse effects and cardiovascular mortality. We conducted quantitative analyses (i.e., meta-analyses) where possible, as described in the Methods chapter. Results of these analyses are presented graphically in the form of forest plots. A list of abbreviations and acronyms used in this chapter is provided at the end of the report.

Results of Literature Searches

Figure 2 depicts the flow of articles through the literature search and screening process. Searches of PubMed®, Embase®, and the Cochrane Database of Systematic Reviews yielded 5769 citations, 756 of which were duplicate citations. Manual searching identified 213 additional citations, for a total of 5226 citations. After applying inclusion/exclusion criteria at the title-and-abstract level, 179 full-text articles were retrieved and screened. Of these, 139 were excluded at the full-text screening stage, leaving 40 articles (representing 35 unique studies) for data abstraction. Note that many articles/studies were relevant to more than one KQ. The information request strategy described in the Methods chapter (contacts to pharmaceutical manufacturers) did not result in any additional data for consideration.

Appendix D provides a detailed listing of included articles. Appendix E provides a complete list of articles excluded at the full-text screening stage, with reasons for exclusion.

Figure 2. Literature flow diagram

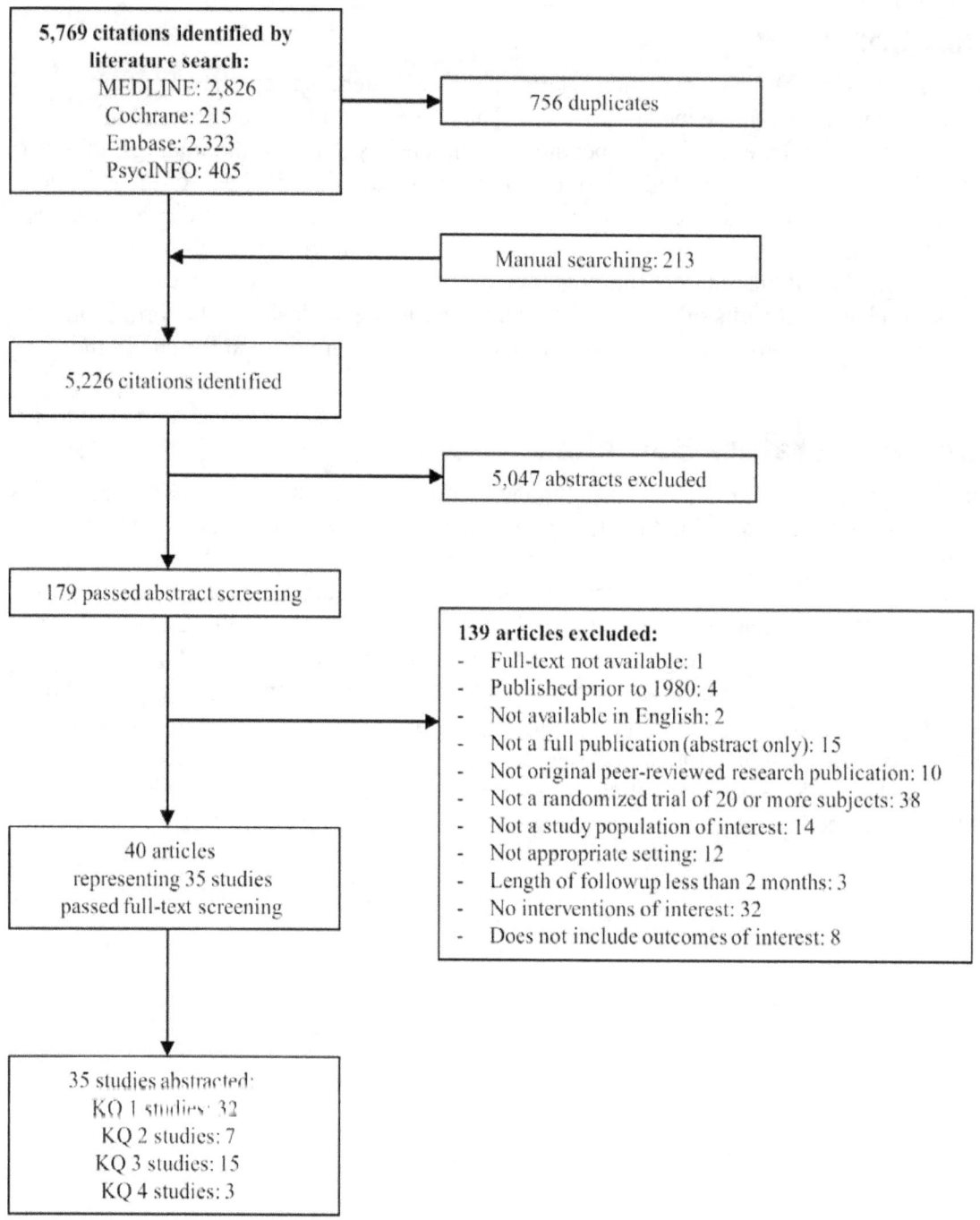

KQ = Key Question

Description of Included Studies

Overall, we included 35 studies, some of which were relevant to more than one KQ: 32 studies were relevant to KQ 1, 7 to KQ 2, 15 to KQ 3, and 3 to KQ 4. Studies were conducted in Europe (23%); Asia (14%); the United States (37%); Australia/New Zealand (6%); and South America (6%); or multiple continents (14%). Sixty-three percent of included studies enrolled individuals with schizophrenia or schizoaffective disorder, eleven percent recruited individuals with schizophrenia, schizoaffective disorder, or bipolar disorder, twenty percent recruited patients either taking antipsychotics or with an unspecified SMI diagnosis, and only six percent recruited individuals with bipolar disorder. The vast majority of studies were specifically designed to control weight (80%); only one study was designed to target diabetes management, and no studies were designed to target dyslipidemia. Table F-1 in Appendix F details the study characteristics for the 35 included studies.

Treatment Network Map

Figure 3 maps the direct comparisons between treatments evaluated in this report. The drugs, treatment indications, and major mechanisms of action are summarized in Table 5. The most common comparisons were between behavioral interventions and control (26% of comparisons), followed by neurologics (13%), and psychotropics or antihistamines compared with control (10% for each comparison). Relatively few studies compared two active interventions. No studies evaluated standard medications for hyperlipidemia (e.g., HMG-CoA reductase inhibitors) or orlistat (a Food and Drug Administration [FDA]-approved medication for weight control), and only a few studies evaluated hypoglycemic medication.

Figure 3. Treatment network describing the number of comparisons for each intervention (35 trials)[a]

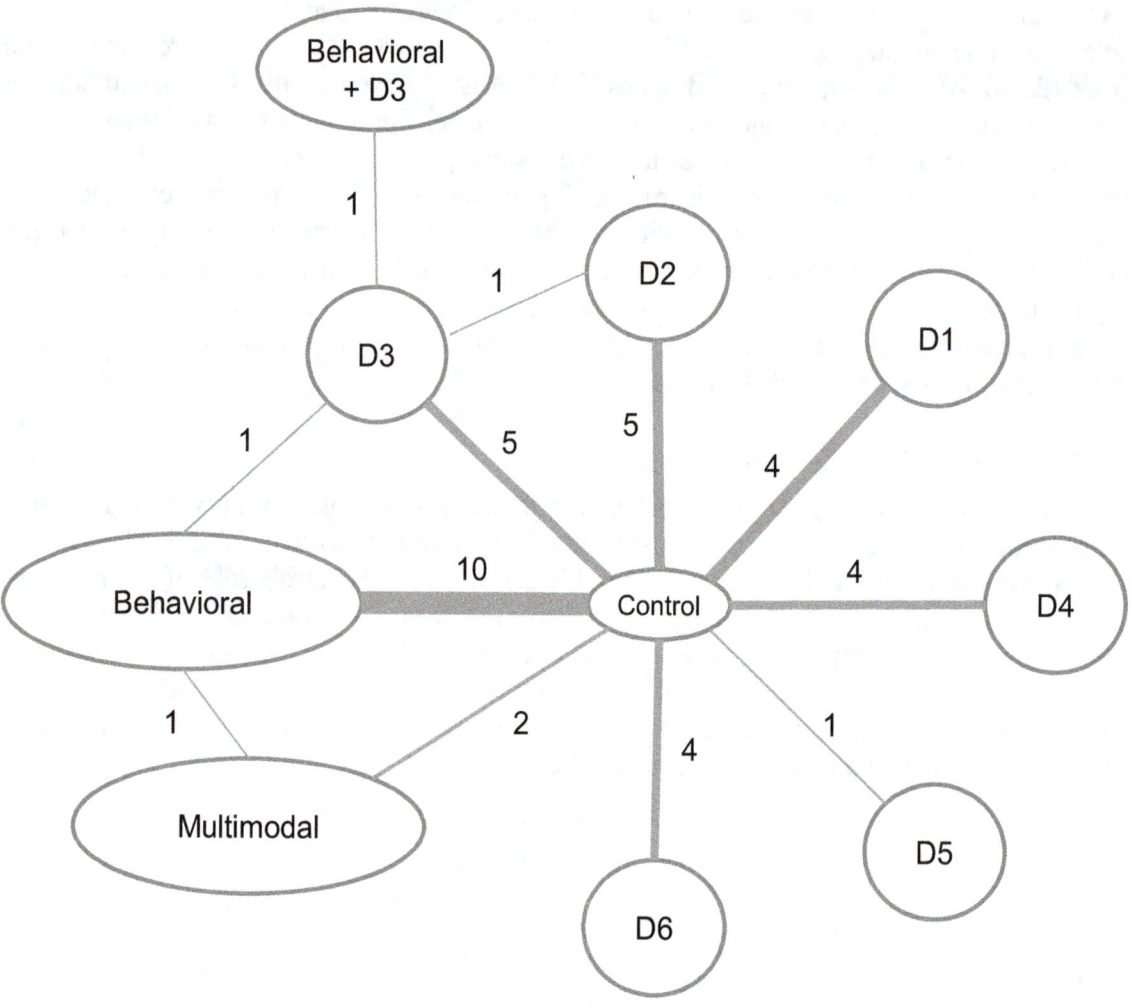

[a]Because some trials had more than two arms, there are more comparisons than trials.
D1 = Psychotropics (aripiprazole, atomoxetine, fluoxetine, ramelteon).
D2 = Neurologics (amantadine, topiramate, zonisamide).
D3=Metformin.
D4 = Antihistamines (nizatidine).
D5 = Nutritionals (carnitine).
D6 = Antipsychotic switching (from oral olanzapine to aripiprazole, olanzapine long-acting injection, olanzapine orally disintegrating).

Drugs Evaluated

Table 5 lists the drugs evaluated in the included studies and their FDA indications and mechanism of action.

Table 5. Drugs evaluated

Drug	FDA Indications	Major Mechanism of Action
Psychotropics		
Atomoxetine	Attention deficit hyperactivity disorder	Selectively inhibits norepinephrine reuptake
Fluoxetine	Major depressive disorder Bipolar disorder Obsessive compulsive disorder Panic disorder Bulimia nervosa	Selectively inhibits serotonin reuptake
Aripiprazole	Schizophrenia Bipolar disorder-manic/mixed Major depressive disorder (adjunctive treatment)	Partially agonizes dopamine D2 and serotonin 5-HT1A receptors, antagonizes serotonin at 5-HT2A receptors
Olanzapine	Schizophrenia Bipolar disorder-depressive Bipolar disorder-manic/mixed Major depressive disorder-treatment resistant	Antagonizes dopamine, serotonin 5-HT2, and other receptors
Quetiapine	Schizophrenia Bipolar disorder-depressive Bipolar disorder-manic Major depressive disorder (adjunctive treatment)	Antagonizes dopamine, serotonin 5-HT2, and other receptors
Ramelteon	Insomnia	Melatonin receptor agonist
Neurologics		
Amantadine	Influenza Extrapyramidal disorders Parkinsonism	Potentiate CNS dopaminergic response; inhibits viral replication
Topiramate	Seizure disorders Migraine prophylaxis	Exact mechanism unknown; blocks sodium channels, increases GABA, antagonizes kainite
Zonisamide	Partial seizures	Exact mechanism unknown; blocks sodium channels and T-type calcium channels, mild carbonic anhydrase inhibiting effects; some augmentation of dopaminergic and serotonergic transmission
Other Drugs		
Metformin	Diabetes mellitus Polycystic ovary syndrome	Decreases hepatic glucose production and intestinal glucose absorption; increases insulin sensitivity
Nizatidine	Duodenal or gastric ulcer treatment Gastroesophageal reflux	Selectively antagonizes histamine H2 receptors
Carnitine	Nutritional (no FDA indication)	Lipid metabolism, lots of studies for many other disease

CNS = central nervous system; FDA = Food and Drug Administration; GABA = gamma-aminobutyric acid

Of the 35 studies, 10 (29%) were judged to be of good quality, 21 (60%) of fair quality, and 4 (11%) of poor quality. Considering individual components of study design and conduct, the strengths were comparable groups at baseline and valid outcome measures. However, 71 percent of studies had inadequate or unclear specification of allocation sequence and concealment, 74 percent had inadequate or unclear specification of protocols for blinding, and 34 percent had high rates of differential attrition. Sixty-six percent of studies were supported at least in part by industry.

Efficacy–Effectiveness Scale

We also categorized studies using an efficacy–effectiveness scale (Appendix B). Studies that have more effectiveness characteristics may be more likely to yield intervention effects that more closely mirror outcomes seen in usual practice. No study was categorized as an effectiveness study. Of the 35 studies, 21 were categorized as efficacy and 14 as mixed efficacy–effectiveness. As shown in Figure 4, the minority of studies were categorized as effectiveness on each of the eight dimensions examined.

Figure 4. Proportion of studies rated as effectiveness studies on each efficacy–effectiveness dimension

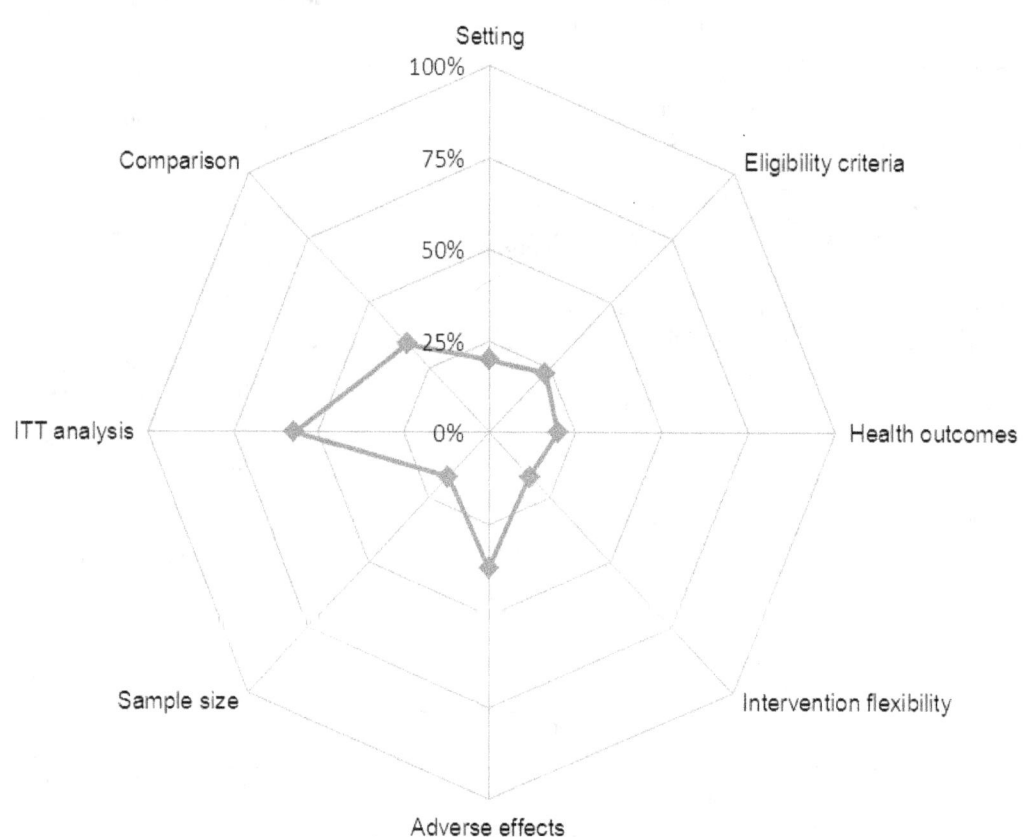

ITT = intention to treat

Further details are provided in the relevant KQ Results sections that follow and in Appendix F, which reports details of the characteristics of each included study, including geographical location, clinical setting, study population, intervention(s), comparator(s), and quality rating.

As described in the Methods chapter, we searched ClinicalTrials.gov to identify completed but unpublished studies as a mechanism for ascertaining publication bias. Our search yielded 1417 citations. A single reviewer identified 73 of these as potentially relevant; 48 of these had been completed at least 1 year prior to our search of the published literature. Of these 48, 18 were published and 4 are among our included studies; 30 had no identified published literature. A total of 25 studies were not completed at least 1 year prior to our search of the published literature. Twenty-four of these are ongoing (10 applicable to KQ 1; 2 applicable to KQ 2; 2 applicable to KQ 3; 3 applicable to KQ 4; 6 applicable to multiple KQs) and 1 was terminated. In summary, our search of ClinicalTrials.gov found evidence for completed but unpublished studies relevant to our KQs.

Key Question 1. Effectiveness of Weight-Management Interventions

KQ 1: What is the effectiveness of weight-management behavioral interventions (e.g., behavioral counseling, health education), peer or family support interventions, pharmacological treatments (e.g., orlistat, topiramate), antipsychotic medication–switching to an antipsychotic with a low or neutral impact on weight, or their combination on weight control and related physical health outcomes (e.g., health-related quality of life, mortality) when compared with each other or with usual care (or other control) among adults with serious mental illness (SMI) who are overweight, obese, or taking antipsychotics?

Key Points

- Of the 32 studies identified, most were specifically designed to control weight gain for individuals with SMI.
- Behavioral interventions were found in a meta-analysis to have a significant advantage over control conditions. We found moderate strength of evidence (SOE) that behavioral interventions are associated with small decreases in weight (about 3 kg) compared with controls.
- Switching to or adding adjunctive aripiprazole, adding the anticonvulsant medications topiramate and zonisamide, or adding metformin yielded small to moderate weight loss (low SOE).
- There was no advantage in favor of nizatidine compared with placebo for the management of weight gain among patients with SMI (low SOE).
- No studies evaluated the weight loss medication orlistat in this population.
- Few studies reported effects on physical functioning or health-related quality of life, and no studies reported all-cause mortality.

Detailed Synthesis

We identified 32 RCTs encompassing 3473 patients that assessed the effects of weight-management strategies among adults with SMI.[88-119] In total, 22 studies targeted weight control,[89-91,93-100,102-104,106,107,109,110,112-114,117,119] 6 obesity prevention,[88,101,111,115,118,119] 3 antipsychotic metabolic effects,[92,108,116] and 1 diabetes management.[105] All identified studies were published from 2003 forward, reflecting the recent clinical interest in weight control among individuals with SMI. Ten trials assessed behavioral intervention strategies compared with control,[88,93,94,97,99,103-105,113,114] 16 assessed pharmacological strategies compared with placebo;[89-92,96,98,100,109-112,115-119] 4 assessed antipsychotic-switching strategies;[95,102,106,108] and 1 four-arm trial assessed metformin alone, lifestyle intervention alone, metformin plus lifestyle intervention, or placebo.[107] Of the 32 trials that reported on weight control, 7 are included in KQ 2 (diabetes control), 14 are included in KQ 3 (dyslipidemia control), and none is included in KQ 4 (multicondition interventions).

Study Characteristics

Table 6 summarizes the study characteristics of the 32 included studies. Most studies (n=19) were rated fair quality, with 9 studies rated good quality and 4 poor quality. Common reasons for reduced study quality were inadequate or unclear specification of the following: allocation sequence and concealment, protocols for blinding of assessments, reported conflicts of interest. We identified no studies rated as effectiveness trials, 20 as efficacy trials, and 12 as mixed efficacy–effectiveness trials. The most common reasons that studies were coded as efficacy trials were because they were conducted in a highly specialized setting, had only short-term followup (<6 months), had inadequate or unspecified sample sizes, or focused on intermediate health outcomes rather than clinically important outcomes. Twelve studies were conducted exclusively with U.S.-based populations. Most studies (n=25) were conducted in outpatient mental health settings. Twenty-one studies received at least partial funding support from industry sponsors.

Of the 3,484 participants across the 32 included studies, most were male and white. Of note, 15 studies did not report race/ethnicity data, and 3 studies did not provide information on the sex of the randomized samples. Twenty-one studies recruited patients with schizophrenia/schizoaffective disorder, three recruited patients with schizophrenia/schizoaffective disorder or bipolar disorder, two recruited participants with bipolar disorder only, and six did not specify psychiatric illness but defined the sample as having SMI or taking antipsychotics. Only 10 studies stated that they recruited participants who were classified as obese or overweight at baseline.

Table 6. Study characteristics for KQ 1: Weight-management interventions

Characteristic	Details
Studies: N (patients)[a]	32 studies (3473 patients)
Mean age of sample: Median (range)	35.5 (25.6 to 53.1)
Sex: N patients (%)	
Female	1353 (39%)
Male	1764 (51%)
NR	356 (10%)
Race: N patients (%)	
White	1568 (45%)
Nonwhite	859 (25%)
NR	1055 (30%)
Baseline weight (kg): Median (range)	81.1 (54.0 to 101.83)
Setting: N studies (%)	
Mental health	25 (78%)
General medical	1 (3%)
Community	2 (6%)
Integrated mental health-medical	0 (0%)
Not reported	4 (13%)
Study quality: N studies (%)[b]	
Good	9 studies (28%)
Fair	19 studies (59%)
Poor	4 studies (13%)
Efficacy–effectiveness rating: N studies (%)	
Efficacy (0–2)	20 studies (63%)
Mixed (3–5)	12 studies (37%)
Effectiveness (6–7)	0 studies (0%)
Comparisons: N studies (patients randomized)	
Drug vs. placebo/control	16 studies (1047 patients)
Antipsychotic vs. antipsychotic switching	4 studies (1520 patients)
Behavioral vs. control	10 studies (662 patients)
Drug vs. behavioral vs. both vs. placebo/control	1 study (128 patients)
Drug vs. drug vs. placebo/control	1 study (199 patients)

kg = kilogram; KQ = Key Question; N = number; NR = not reported
[a]The number of patients with demographic data reported is fewer than the number randomized.
[b]Quality ratings in the table are reported on the basis of how studies were conducted in relation to laboratory-based physical health outcomes. Ratings were also applied on the basis of patient-reported outcomes. Only one quality rating differed on the basis of physical versus patient-reported outcomes[103] and was rated as fair on laboratory-based physical health outcomes and poor on patient-reported outcomes.

Meta-Analysis and Qualitative Review

We classified studies and organized findings by the following intervention categories: (1) behavioral interventions, (2) peer or family support interventions, (3) pharmacological treatments (psychotropic agents [e.g., atomoxetine, aripiprazole, fluoxetine], neurologic agents [e.g., topiramate, amantadine, zonisamide], metformin, nizatidine, and carnitine), and (4) antipsychotic-switching interventions.

We had sufficient studies to perform four meta-analyses. The other comparisons were synthesized qualitatively. Below, we focus on the weight control outcomes and, when reported, adverse effects (i.e., discontinuation due to adverse effects, significant worsening of psychiatric symptoms), and health-related quality of life. While mortality was an outcome of interest, no study reported on this outcome. Details for HbA1c are in the Results section of KQ 2, and details for lipids are in KQ 3.

Effect of Behavioral Interventions on Weight Control

Eleven studies, 3 rated good quality,[88,104,107] 6 fair,[93,94,99,103,105,113] and 2 poor,[97,114] measured the impact of behavioral interventions on weight control among individuals with SMI. As expected, most patients also were on antipsychotics or mood stabilizers at baseline and continued these medications throughout the intervention. The median baseline weight across these studies was 83.9 kg (range, 64.6 to 101.8 kg). The number of treatment sessions ranged from 4 to 24 and the treatment duration ranged from 8 weeks to 6 months. Six of these studies were classified as more intensive behavioral strategies, operationalized as at least six contacts over 12 weeks, a written manual of counseling protocol, and skills-based versus education-based intervention content. Interventions were adapted for SMI populations by streamlining content to focus on key points, delivery of intervention content by mental health personnel, and use of specific behavior change strategies (e.g., goal setting, modeling, healthy food sampling), and incorporating psychoeducation about SMI. Control conditions consisted of waitlist, no intervention, and usual care plus information. These control group conditions were combined in the meta-analysis, as participants in waitlist and no intervention conditions were allowed to continue receiving usual care. Selected details of each intervention are in Table 7.

Table 7. Details of behavioral interventions

Citation	Planned Contacts	Written Manual?	Strategies Used
Alvarez-Jimenez, 2006[88]	10 to 14 weekly or twice-weekly individual therapy sessions over 3 months	Yes	Education about diet and physical activity Problem solving Goal setting Motivational techniques Self-monitoring Activity scheduling Personalized or tailored written communications
Brar, 2005[93]	20 behavioral therapy sessions, twice weekly for 6 weeks followed by weekly for 8 weeks	Yes	Education about diet and physical activity Self-monitoring Cognitive and behavioral approaches to reduce overeating
Brown, 2011[94]	12 weekly individual visits followed by monthly individual visits and weekly phone calls for the following 3 months	Yes	Education about diet and physical activity Problem solving Goal setting Activity scheduling Strategies to enhance social support Meal replacements
Evans, 2005[97]	6 individual nutrition education sessions over 3 months	No	Education about diet and physical activity Goal setting
Gillhoff, 2010[99]	Weekly fitness training, 7 psychotherapeutic/educational sessions, and 4 cooking and nutrition classes over the course of 5 months.	No	Patient psychoeducation about bipolar disorders Education about diet and physical activity Goal setting Motivational techniques Activity scheduling Stress management techniques
Khazaal, 2007[113]	12 weekly CBT-based group sessions over 6 months	Yes	Education about diet and physical activity Psychoeducation about links between weight gain and antipsychotic drugs Self-monitoring Meal tastings

Table 7. Details of behavioral interventions (continued)

Citation	Planned Contacts	Written Manual?	Strategies Used
Kwon, 2006[103]	8 individual sessions of CBT weight management counseling over 3 months	No	Education about diet and physical activity Problem-solving skills Goal setting Self-monitoring Activity scheduling
Littrell, 2003[104]	16 weekly 1-hour classes over 4 months	Yes	Education about diet and physical activity Goal setting Self-monitoring Activity scheduling Strategies to enhance social support
Mauri, 2008[114]	5 to 7 psychoeducational groups over 4 months	No	Education about diet and physical activity Goal setting Self-monitoring Personalized or tailored written communications Education on controlling stimuli to overeat
McKibbin, 2006[105]	24 weekly 90-minute group classes over 6 months	Yes	Education about diet and physical activity Diabetes education Self-monitoring Reinforcements (i.e., raffle tickets for small health-related prizes) Behavioral modeling Skills practice
Wu, 2008[107]	4 psychoeducational session and 7 sessions with an exercise physiologist (during the first week only) and consultation with a dietitian (frequency not stated) over 3 months	No	Education about diet and physical activity Education about monitoring adherence with family member/caregiver Goal setting Self-monitoring Activity scheduling Personalized or tailored written communications Homework assignments

CBT = cognitive behavioral therapy

Of these 11 studies, one assessed weight control only as a change in BMI and could not be combined with the other studies that assessed weight control as a change in kilograms or pounds;[105] this study is discussed in detail in the KQ 2 section. In brief, the study found that participants in the behavioral intervention group experienced greater improvements in BMI from baseline to 12-month followup compared with usual care (approximately -1 vs. +0.05 BMI points, p<0.01).

Figure 5 shows the forest plot of the meta-analysis examining the effect of behavioral interventions compared with control on weight gain, which included the remaining 10 studies (735 participants).[88,93,94,97,99,103,104,107,113,114] In these studies, the behavioral intervention led to a mean difference of -3.13 kg (95% CI, -4.21 to -2.05), an effect of small magnitude (approximately 4% reduction in body weight over baseline). In an exploratory subgroup analysis by intervention intensity, high-intensity behavioral intervention resulted in a mean difference of -2.43 kg compared with control (CI, -4.23 to -0.62). There was some evidence of moderate heterogeneity (Q-value=10.428, df=4, p=0.034; I^2=61.643). Low-intensity behavioral intervention resulted in a mean difference of -3.53 kg weight compared with control (CI, -4.88 to -2.17). There was some evidence of low heterogeneity as assessed by the I^2 value of 34.925 but no evidence of heterogeneity as assessed by the Q-value of 6.147 for 4 degrees of freedom (p=0.188). There was no significant difference between low- and high-intensity behavioral interventions (chi-square=0.91, df=1, p=0.34). Analyses were repeated excluding the two studies rated as poor quality.[97,114] These exclusions had a minor effect on the odds ratio estimates for all studies combined (-3.10 kg; CI, -4.65 to -1.54).

Figure 5. Forest plot of meta-analysis of effect of behavioral interventions on weight

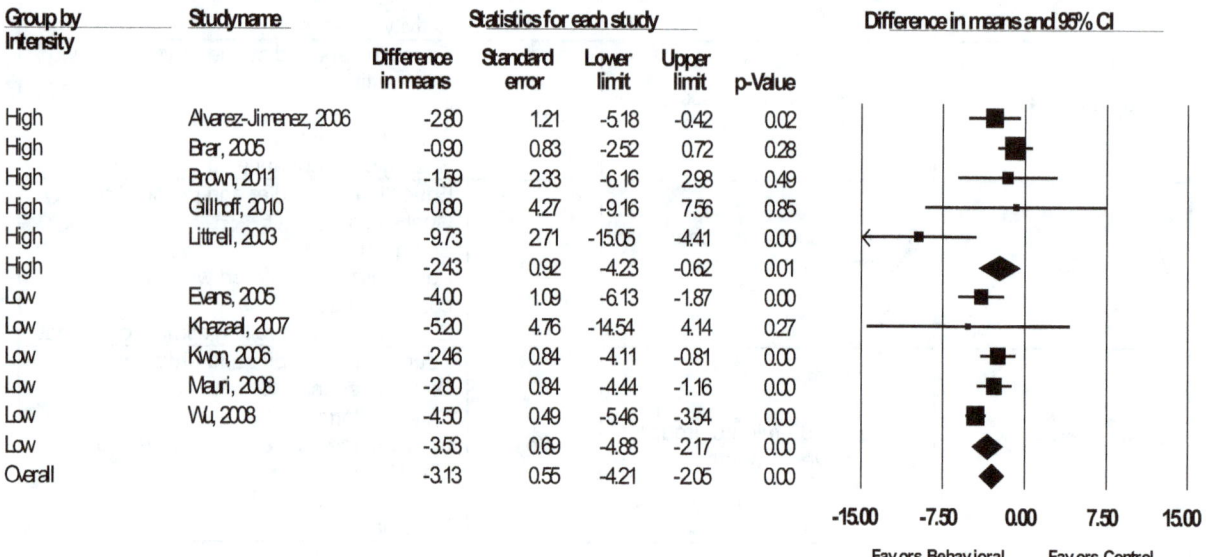

Group by Intensity	Study name	Difference in means	Standard error	Lower limit	Upper limit	p-Value	Difference in means and 95% CI
High	Alvarez-Jimenez, 2006	-2.80	1.21	-5.18	-0.42	0.02	
High	Brar, 2005	-0.90	0.83	-2.52	0.72	0.28	
High	Brown, 2011	-1.59	2.33	-6.16	2.98	0.49	
High	Gillhoff, 2010	-0.80	4.27	-9.16	7.56	0.85	
High	Littrell, 2003	-9.73	2.71	-15.05	-4.41	0.00	
High		-2.43	0.92	-4.23	-0.62	0.01	
Low	Evans, 2005	-4.00	1.09	-6.13	-1.87	0.00	
Low	Khazaal, 2007	-5.20	4.76	-14.54	4.14	0.27	
Low	Kwon, 2006	-2.46	0.84	-4.11	-0.81	0.00	
Low	Mauri, 2008	-2.80	0.84	-4.44	-1.16	0.00	
Low	Wu, 2008	-4.50	0.49	-5.46	-3.54	0.00	
Low		-3.53	0.69	-4.88	-2.17	0.00	
Overall		-3.13	0.55	-4.21	-2.05	0.00	

CI = confidence interval

For the studies that reported adverse effects, none reported significant differences between conditions in serious adverse effects as defined by the study protocol, and only three studies[93,105,107] reported discontinuations due to serious or nonserious adverse effects and found no difference between groups. One study reported health-related quality of life,[103] assessing physical health status with the World Health Organization-Quality of Life Brief Version instrument, and found no significant differences between behavioral weight management and control. Funnel plots for publication bias did not demonstrate evidence of publication bias.

Effect of Peer or Family Support Interventions on Weight Control

We identified no eligible studies for this category of intervention for KQ 1.

Effect of Pharmacological Treatments on Weight Control

Psychotropic Agents

Four studies, 1 rated good quality[98] and 3 fair,[91,92,109] assessed the impact of psychotropic agents atomoxetine,[91] fluoxetine,[109] aripiprazole,[98] and ramelteon[92] on weight control among second-generation antipsychotic-treated individuals with schizophrenia. Although each medication is classified as psychotropic, the mechanisms of action vary. Thus, we did not perform a meta-analysis; instead, key findings are synthesized qualitatively.

Across included studies, participants treated with psychotropic agents experienced variable levels of weight control on the four medications. For participants who lost weight, effects were modest (range, -0.15 to -2.53 kg), which translates into less than 3 percent change in body weight from baseline (median baseline weight, 81.5 kg; range, 80.5 to 102.2 kg). Only one study demonstrated significant weight loss; this study was also the only one that reported discontinuation due to side effects and health-related quality of life outcomes.[98]

A good-quality study[98] assessed weight gain in clozapine-treated outpatients with schizophrenia (207 patients). First, patients on a fixed dose of clozapine (200 to 900 mg/day) were randomized to an adjunctive flexible dose of aripiprazole (5 to 15 mg/day) or clozapine plus placebo. After 16 weeks, patients who completed the 16-week double blind phase could enter a 12-week open-label extension phase. All patients received 5 to 15 mg per day of aripiprazole and flexible dosing of clozapine. At 16 weeks, adjunctive aripiprazole significantly decreased weight compared with placebo control (-2.53 vs. -0.38 kg, $p<0.001$). A total of 180 participants entered the 12-week open-label phase in which everyone received adjunctive aripiprazole. Participants originally randomized to adjunctive aripiprazole continued to lose weight and, at the end, experienced a mean change in weight of -3.26 kg from baseline weight. Those who had originally received placebo had a -1.88 kg mean weight loss over the 12-week open-label phase. Treatment with adjunctive aripiprazole did not differentially impact health-related quality of life compared with placebo control as measured by the Subjective Well Being Under Neuroleptics scale ($p=0.20$). Only one participant in the placebo arm and five in the aripiprazole arm discontinued the trial due to adverse effects. However, 0 out of 99 patients in the placebo group and 10 out of 108 patients in the aripiprazole group experienced a serious adverse effect.

In another study rated fair quality,[91] 37 olanzapine- or clozapine-treated individuals with schizophrenia were randomized to 24 weeks of either atomoxetine or placebo. Atomoxetine was titrated from 40 mg per day to 120 mg per day, which is above the normal recommended dosage. All participants also received a diet and exercise program that consisted of 10 weeks of a Weight Watchers program and exercise sessions three times per week. Participants could receive tokens for compliance with exercise and diet programs; tokens could be used to acquire prizes at the end of the study. Both atomoxetine and placebo groups lost weight; however, results were modest and not significant (-1.7 kg vs. -2.1 kg, $p=0.82$). Adherence to the exercise and diet program was low; only nine participants who completed the study also adhered to the program. However, these nine participants lost more weight (range, -15.9 to -4.5 kg).

In a fair-quality study of olanzapine-treated schizophrenic patients,[109] patients who had gained at least 3 percent over baseline weight were randomized to a double-blind 4-month treatment of placebo or fluoxetine (20 to 60 mg/day). During the olanzapine-only phase, two patients were hospitalized for worsening of psychiatric symptoms, and one died for causes deemed unrelated to the study. Fifty-one patients started on olanzapine and 31 met weight-gain criteria for randomization to fluoxetine or placebo with continued treatment on olanzapine. Both groups gained weight. The fluoxetine-treated patients did not gain less weight than the placebo controls ($p=0.3$).

In a small, double-blind, 8-week trial rated fair quality,[92] 20 participants with schizophrenia were randomized to adjunctive ramelteon (8 mg/day) or placebo. All patients entered the study on second-generation antipsychotics and were maintained on these during the trial. Patients on ramelteon did not experience significant weight loss compared with placebo control (-0.84 vs. -0.15, $p=0.28$).

Neurologic Agents

Four studies, 1 rated good quality,[115] 2 fair,[112,119] and 1 poor,[100] assessed the effects of neurologic agents topiramate, amantadine, or zonisamide on weight control among individuals with SMI treated with olanzapine. One study was conducted with women only.[112] Two were conducted with participants with schizophrenia,[100,119] one with an SMI population on olanzapine,[112] and one with a mixed population of people with psychotic or bipolar disorder.[115] Three studies assessed anticonvulsant medications topiramate[112,119] and zonisamide[115] versus placebo control on the effects of olanzapine-induced weight gain; these studies were able to be combined in a meta-analysis (Figure 6). Results for the amantadine placebo-controlled trial are summarized qualitatively.

Figure 6 shows the forest plot of the meta-analysis examining the effect of anticonvulsant medications compared with placebo control on olanzapine-induced weight gain, which included 3 studies (158 participants) (median baseline weight, 86.6 kg; range, 54.0 to 95.6 kg). The analysis demonstrated statistically significant difference in efficacy between topiramate and zonisamide versus placebo control on weight gain of -5.11 kg (95% CI, -9.48 to -0.74), a clinically significant weight loss of a small effect (approximately 6% reduction in body weight over baseline compared with median baseline weight). There was no evidence of heterogeneity (Q-value=0.332, df =2, p=0.733; I^2=0.000).

Figure 6. Forest plot of meta-analysis of effect of anticonvulsant medications topiramate and zonisamide on weight

Study name	Statistics for each study					Difference in means and 95% CI
	Difference in means	Standard error	Lower limit	Upper limit	p-Value	
McElroy, 2012	-4.30	8.80	-21.54	12.94	0.63	
Narula, 2010	-6.12	3.18	-12.35	0.11	0.05	
Nickel, 2005	-4.10	3.36	-10.68	2.48	0.22	
	-5.11	2.23	-9.48	-0.74	0.02	

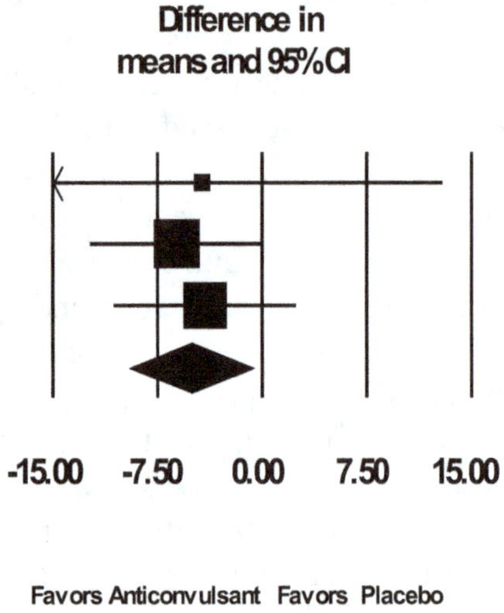

-15.00   -7.50   0.00   7.50   15.00

Favors Anticonvulsant   Favors Placebo

CI = confidence interval

Results of the single amantadine study mirror these findings.[100] This 12-week study of amantadine versus placebo among 21 SMI patients who had gained at least 5 pounds on olanzapine also found significant but small improvements with adjunctive amantadine (-0.7 vs. +1.24 kg/m^2).

One study[112] reported on health-related quality of life; participants taking olanzapine and randomized to adjunctive topiramate had significant improvements on seven of eight scales of SF-36 compared with adjunctive placebo control. Two studies reported on discontinuation from the studies for adverse effects.[100,115] One patient randomized to amantadine withdrew from the study due to significant worsening of psychosis.[100] Ten participants in the placebo-controlled study of zonisamide[115] withdrew from the study for adverse effects (five in placebo group and five in zonisamide group). Because formal statistical techniques for publication bias are not effective with small numbers of studies, we did not conduct analyses for publication bias.

Metformin

Five studies, two rated good quality,[107,118] two fair,[116,117] and one poor,[101] assessed the effects of metformin on weight control for individuals with SMI. All studies were conducted with participants with schizophrenia; three trials were conducted solely with first-psychotic-episode participants.[107,117,118] All patients were stable on antipsychotics at baseline and continued use of baseline antipsychotics during the trial. Four of these studies[107,116-118] assessed metformin versus placebo control; these studies were able to be combined in a meta-analysis (Figure 7). The final study[101] compared three different treatment algorithms; results of this trial are summarized qualitatively.

Figure 7 shows the forest plot of the meta-analysis examining the effect of metformin compared with placebo control on weight gain that included 332 participants (median baseline weight, 64.7 kg; range, 64.8 to 79.4 kg). The analysis demonstrated statistically significant difference in efficacy between metformin versus placebo on weight gain of -4.13 kg (95% CI, -6.58 to -1.68), a clinically significant difference of a small effect (percentage of body weight lost from baseline range, 5% to 6%). There was evidence of extreme heterogeneity (Q value=32,318, 3 df, $p < 0.001$; I^2=90.717).

Figure 7. Forest plot of meta-analysis of effect of metformin on weight

Study name	Statistics for each study					Difference in means and 95% CI
	Difference in means	Standard error	Lower limit	Upper limit	p-Value	
Carrizo, 2009	-2.03	0.79	-3.59	-0.47	0.01	
Wang, 2012	-5.00	1.37	-7.69	-2.31	0.00	
Wu, 2008	-6.30	0.51	-7.29	-5.31	0.00	
Wu, 2012	-3.02	1.32	-5.60	-0.44	0.02	
	-4.13	1.25	-6.58	-1.68	0.00	

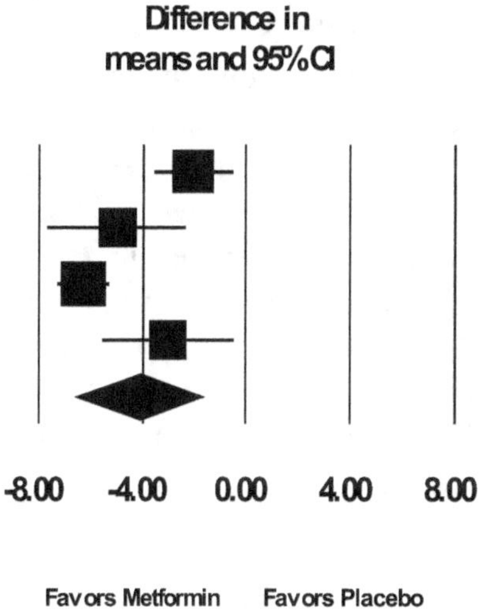

-8.00   -4.00   0.00   4.00   8.00

Favors Metformin   Favors Placebo

CI = confidence interval

In a poor-quality study, Hoffmann et al.[101] randomly assigned 199 nondiabetic outpatients with schizophrenia or schizoaffective disorder to 1 of 3 conditions for 22 weeks: (1) olanzapine only, (2) olanzapine plus 200 mg/day amantadine with possible switches to 1000 to 1500 mg/day metformin and then switches to 100 to 400 mg/day zonisamide (treatment algorithm A), or (3) olanzapine plus 1000 to 1500 mg/day metformin with possible switches to 200 mg/day amantadine and then switches to 100 to 400 mg/day zonisamide (treatment algorithm B). Forty-two percent of participants of algorithm A and 35 percent of algorithm B switched to second treatment. The estimated time to switching to second treatment for 25 percent of the sample was 42 days for algorithm A and 66 days for algorithm B. A combined treatment group of both algorithm A and algorithm B did not differ significantly from the olanzapine-only group at 22-week followup (results not reported, p=0.065). However, patients treated with algorithm B compared with olanzapine-only resulted in significantly less weight gain (0.65 vs. 2.76 kg, p=0.04), though the magnitude of the effect was small. Ten subjects continued the study despite serious adverse effects (1 in algorithm A group, 4 in algorithm B group, and 5 in olanzapine only group).

None of these studies reported on health-related quality of life. Four of these studies[101,107,117,118] reported on discontinuation from the studies for adverse effects. Among the trials that compared metformin with placebo, no significant differences between conditions were reported across three studies.[107,117,118] In total, 14 participants discontinued the drug due to adverse effects (8 in algorithm A group, 4 in algorithm B group, and 2 in olanzapine only group); only three of these, all in the algorithm A group, were considered serious adverse effects.[101] Because formal statistical techniques for publication bias are not effective with small numbers of studies, we did not conduct analyses for publication bias.

Nizatidine

Four studies, one rated good quality[89] and three fair,[90,110,111] assessed the effects of nizatidine, a histamine2 (H2)-receptor antagonist, on antipsychotic-induced weight gain among people with schizophrenia. One studied assessed weight gain among quetiapine-treated patients[90] while the remaining studies focused on weight gain among olanzapine-treated patients.[89,110,111] Three studies tested nizatidine at recommended therapeutic doses of 300 mg/day;[90,110,111] one study assessed nizatidine at twice the recommended daily dose.[89] Below, we focus on the weight and adverse effects outcomes of these studies.

Figure 8 shows the forest plot of the meta-analysis examining the effect of nizatidine compared with placebo control on antipsychotic-induced weight gain, which included 4 studies (286 participants). The estimated effect shows that nizatidine resulted in a -0.49 kg weight gain compared with placebo that was not statically significant (95% CI, -1.26 to 0.27). There was no evidence of heterogeneity (Q-value =3.030, df=3, p=0.387). However, the I^2 value displayed high heterogeneity (I^2 =0.98). Only one study reported discontinuation due to adverse events; Assuncao et al.[89] reported three patients discontinued the study due to adverse effects (two in the nizatidine treated group). No studies reported on health-related quality of life outcomes. Because formal statistical techniques for publication bias are not effective with small numbers of studies, we did not conduct analyses for publication bias.

Figure 8. Forest plot of meta-analysis of effect of nizatidine on weight

Study name	Statistics for each study					Difference in means and 95% CI
	Difference in means	Standard error	Lower limit	Upper limit	p-Value	
Assuncao, 2006	0.90	6.95	-12.72	14.52	0.90	
Atmaco, 2004	-3.10	1.73	-6.49	0.29	0.07	
Atmaca, 2003	-7.50	9.40	-25.93	10.93	0.43	
Cavazzoni, 2003	-0.35	0.34	-1.02	0.32	0.31	
	-0.49	0.39	-1.26	0.27	0.20	

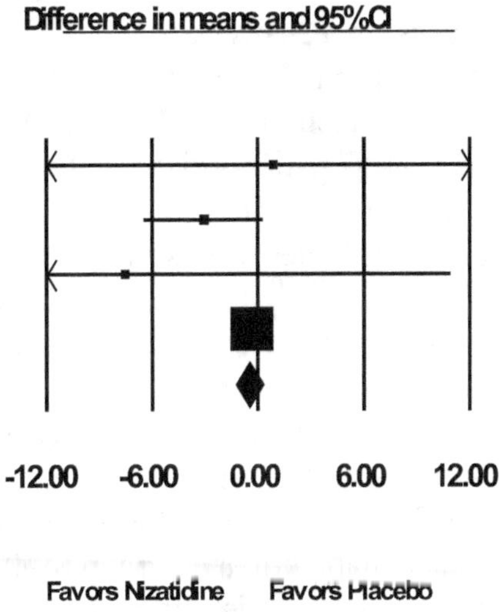

-12.00   -6.00   0.00   6.00   12.00

Favors Nizatidine   Favors Placebo

CI = confidence interval

Carnitine

One good-quality study[96] assessed the effects of 15 mg/kg daily carnitine, a nutritional supplement, compared with placebo among 60 bipolar patients taking sodium valproate for 26 weeks. All study participants also were on energy-restricted, lowfat diets (-500 kcal/day from usual consumption). There is no recommended dose of carnitine; dosages vary and several doses have been studied in scientific research (50 to 100 mg/kg/day, 2 to 6 grams daily, 990 mg two to three times per day). Carnitine had no significant effect on mean weight loss in the study compared with placebo (-1.9 kg vs. -0.9 kg, p=0.38). No other outcomes of interest were reported.

Effect of Antipsychotic-Switching Interventions on Weight Control

Four studies, one rated good quality[102] and three fair,[95,106,108] assessed the effects of antipsychotic-switching strategies on weight control. Patients in all studies began on olanzapine, with the control group maintained on olanzapine. The intervention in two studies involved switching to a different form of olanzapine (an orally disintegrating tablet[102] or a long-acting injection[108]) and in the other two studies, switching to a different antipsychotic medication, quetiapine[95] or aripiprazole.[106] Meta-analysis was not completed on these four studies due to the heterogeneity of switching strategies. Only one study reported on health-related quality of life outcomes. Results are summarized qualitatively.

Neither study that examined switching to a different form of olanzapine[102,108] showed significant effects on weight control. In a good-quality study of a 16-week trial with SMI patients (n=149) that involved switching from 5 to 20 mg of standard olanzapine tablets (SOT) to 5 to 20 mg orally disintegrating olanzapine (ODO) tablets,[102] there was no difference between SOT or ODO groups for mean weight gain (+2.08 vs. +1.42, p=0.39). Results for health-related quality of life as measured by the Subjective Well-being Under Neuroleptics Scale showed no significant change from baseline to followup between groups (p=0.16). Two patients in each group discontinued treatment due to adverse effects. Two patients in the ODO group experienced a serious adverse effect.

Another fair-quality study assessed switching from 10 to 20 mg of oral olanzapine to a long-acting intramuscular injection of olanzapine (150 mg/2 weeks, 405 mg/4 weeks or 300 mg/2 weeks) in a 24-week trial of 921 patients with schizophrenia.[108] Patients taking both formulations of olanzapine experienced statistically significant increases in weight compared with baseline (+1.3 [injection] vs. +1.3 [oral]). However, there were no between-group differences (p=0.34). A total of 57 patients discontinued use due to adverse effects, but there were no differences between groups (p-value NR).

The studies that examined switching from olanzapine to a different antipsychotic medication[95,106] had mixed results. In a fair-quality study, 133 overweight patients with schizophrenia were either switched to 300 to 800 mg/day of quetiapine or continued on 7.5 to 20 mg/day olanzapine.[95] Treatment continued for 24 weeks. Mean weight change between olanzapine and quetiapine were not significant (+0.99 vs. -0.82, p=0.089). Significantly more subjects in the olanzapine group completed 24 weeks of treatment than the quetiapine group (70.3% vs. 43. 1%, p=0.002). Discontinuation due to psychiatric adverse effects was higher in the quetiapine-treated group (p=0.003). However, no significant differences were observed for nonpsychiatric discontinuations (p-value NR). There were no significant differences in hospitalization rates (7.69% in the quetiapine group vs. 1.47% in the olanzapine group, p-value not reported). No other serious adverse events were reported.

In a fair-quality study, 173 patients with schizophrenia either stayed on 10 to 20 mg of olanzapine or switched to 10 to 30mg of aripiprazole in a 16-week trial.[106] Patients who switched to aripiprazole experienced significantly more weight loss than those remaining on olanzapine (-1.84 vs. +1.31 kg, p=0.001), a difference of small magnitude between groups. A total of 15 participants discontinued treatment due to adverse effects (7 aripiprazole-treated, 8 olanzapine-treated). Six participants treated with aripiprazole experienced a serious adverse effect compared with nine in the olanzapine-treated group (p-value NR). Another study, described in KQ 4, evaluated switching to aripiprazole as part of a multicomponent intervention.[120] This study found that patients who switched to aripiprazole lost more weight than those who stayed on their current antipsychotic medication. (See KQ 4 section for more details.)

Summary of Key Question 1

Overall, only 9 of the 32 trials identified as relevant for KQ 1 were of good quality. Thus, the majority of studies had important design or reporting deficits. Most trials were specifically designed to control weight gain for individuals with SMI. Other studies targeted diabetes management or antipsychotic metabolic effects but also reported effects on weight management. The 32 trials assessed the impact of a wide variety of pharmacological and behavioral strategies on weight among individuals with SMI. However, most of the pharmacological strategies assessed in the included interventions were used in treatment of individuals with mental illnesses; no studies evaluated the weight loss medication orlistat in this population. The behavioral interventions, anticonvulsant agents topiramate and zonisamide, and metformin were associated with greater weight loss than controls (for behavioral interventions) or placebo (for pharmacological agents), but the effects were modest. Using adjunctive aripiprazole or switching to aripiprazole also showed promise. Again, the magnitude of effects was small. Discontinuation due to adverse effects and worsening of psychiatric symptoms were not consistently reported. Few studies reported effects on physical functioning or health-related quality of life, and no studies reported cardiovascular mortality.

Key Question 2. Effectiveness of Diabetes-Management Interventions

KQ 2: What is the effectiveness of diabetes-management behavioral interventions (e.g., behavioral counseling, health education), peer or family support interventions, pharmacological treatments (e.g., rosiglitazone, metformin), antipsychotic medication–switching to an antipsychotic with a low or neutral impact on glucose level, or their combination on glucose-level control and related physical health outcomes (e.g., health-related quality of life, mortality) when compared with each other or with usual care (or other control) among adults with SMI who have diabetes or are taking antipsychotics?

Key Points

- Overall, we found insufficient evidence to support any strategy to control glucose. Of the seven studies identified, only one evaluated an intervention specifically designed to target glucose control in individuals with SMI who have diabetes. Two additional studies evaluated interventions targeting nondiabetic individuals who had or were at risk for poor glycemic control. Four studies evaluated interventions targeting weight, with glycemic control as a secondary outcome.
- The interventions represented in these seven studies were ramelteon, antipsychotic switching, metformin, amantadine, and behavioral interventions.
- Just two of the trials found significant advantages for the intervention in controlling HbA1c, with both of these studies involving the use of metformin. Improvements in HbA1c were small.
- Health-related quality of life and serious adverse events were inconsistently reported in the seven trials. Only one study reported effects on physical functioning or health-related quality of life, and no studies reported cardiovascular mortality.

Detailed Synthesis

Of the seven studies identified as relevant to KQ 2 (681 participants),[92,95,99,101,102,105,116] only one study[105] tested an intervention intended specifically for individuals with diabetes mellitus. Two studies[92,116] targeted antipsychotic-induced metabolic risks, including glycemic control as measured by HbA1c, and four studies[95,99,101,102] targeted weight, with HbA1c as a secondary outcome. Of the seven trials that reported on HbA1c, all were included in KQ 1 (weight control), 6 were included in KQ 3 (lipid control), and none were included in KQ 4 (multicondition interventions). All identified studies were published from 2006 forward, reflecting the recent clinical interest in glycemic control among people with SMI.

Study Characteristics

Table 8 summarizes the study characteristics of the seven included studies. Of these, one study was rated good quality,[102] five fair,[92,95,99,105,116] and one poor.[101] Common reasons for reduced study quality were inadequate reporting of randomization and concealment and recruiting procedures, lack of clarity about blinding of outcome assessors, and some difficulties implementing the study protocols as intended.

We identified no effectiveness studies, four efficacy studies,[92,99,105,116] and three studies assessed in the mixed range on the efficacy–effectiveness continuum.[95,101,102] Three studies were conducted exclusively with U.S.-based populations, one was conducted in Europe, and three were conducted in multiple countries. Indicative of care patterns for this population, most studies were conducted in outpatient mental health settings. Trials were funded by private industries (n=4), government (n=1), or a combination of industry and government sources (n=2).

The intervention strategies assessed in these seven studies were the psychotropic medication ramelteon (one study[92]), antipsychotic switching (two studies[95,102]), metformin (two studies[101,116]), and behavioral interventions (two studies[99,105]). All five studies that primarily employed medications as the intervention strategy[92,95,101,102,116] required participants to be on antipsychotic medications at baseline. Of the two behavioral interventions, one required use of a defined group of mood stabilizers (including some antipsychotic medications, some anticonvulsant mood stabilizers, and lithium)[99] and one had no requirement for entry based on medication use.[105]

A total of 681 participants were randomized in the seven studies, ranging from 20 to 199 participants. Most patients were middle-aged and white. Two studies representing 29.0 percent of the overall participants for KQ 2[95,116] did not report sex. In the five studies that reported sex, males outnumbered females 59 to 41 percent. Five studies recruited individuals with schizophrenia or schizoaffective disorder,[92,95,101,105,116] one included individuals with bipolar disorder,[99] and one included individuals with any of these three diagnoses or another related psychotic disorder.[102] Only one study recruited patients with a diagnosis of diabetes.[105] In this study, the mean A1c was 7.0 at baseline, indicating fair glycemic control. Across all included studies, median baseline HbA1c was 5.6 (range, 5.4 to 7.0).

Table 8. Study characteristics for KQ 2: Diabetes-management interventions

Characteristic	Details
Studies: N (patients)[a]	7 studies (681 patients)
Mean baseline HbA1c: Median (range)	5.6 (5.4 to 7.0)
Mean age of sample: Median (range)	44.0 (38.5 to 54.0)
Sex: N patients (%) Female Male NR	197 patients (29%) 278 patients (42%) 194 patients (29%)
Race: N patients (%) White Nonwhite NR	222 patients (35%) 233 patients (37%) 183 patients (28%)
Setting: N studies (%) Mental health General medical Community Integrated mental health-medical Not reported	4 studies (57%) 0 study (0%) 2 studies (29%) 0 studies (0%) 1 study (14%)

Table 8. Study characteristics for KQ 2: Diabetes-management interventions (continued)

Characteristic	Details

Study quality: N studies (%)[b]
  Good
  Fair
  Poor
	1 study (14%)
	5 studies (71%)
	1 study (14%)

Efficacy–effectiveness rating: N studies (%)
  Efficacy (0–2)
  Mixed (3–5)
  Effectiveness (6–7)
	4 studies (57%)
	3 studies (43%)
	0 studies (0%)

Comparisons: N studies (patients randomized)
  Drug vs. placebo/control
  Antipsychotic switching vs. antipsychotic stay
  Behavioral vs. control
  Drug vs. drug vs. placebo/control
	2 studies (81 patients)
	2 studies (282 patients)
	2 studies (114 patients)
	1 study (199 patients)

N = number; NR = not reported

[a]The number of patients with demographic data reported is fewer than the number randomized.

[b]Quality ratings in the table are reported on the basis of how studies were conducted in relation to laboratory-based physical health outcomes. Ratings were also applied on the basis of patient-reported outcomes. Raters were the same as for laboratory-based outcomes except that two studies[92,99] did not report patient-reported outcomes.

Qualitative Review

HbA1c is the most consistently reported measure of glycemic control in these studies and is a widely accepted and reliable measure; therefore, we used it as the outcome measure for glycemic control for this evidence synthesis. There was an insufficient number of studies to conduct meta-analyses on the effects of any of the intervention classes by HbA1c. Results are summarized qualitatively. We focus on the HbA1c outcomes and, when reported, adverse effects (i.e. discontinuation due to adverse events, significant worsening of psychiatric symptoms). While health-related quality of life and mortality were outcomes of interest, only one study reported on health-related quality of life, and no studies reported on mortality. Details for weight and lipids can be found in KQ 1 and KQ 3, respectively. Also, because formal statistical techniques for publication bias are not effective with small numbers of studies, we did not conduct analyses for publication bias.

Effect of Behavioral Interventions on Diabetes Control

Two studies evaluated behavioral interventions, one specifically designed to target diabetes[105] and one with the primary target of weight with glycemic control measured as a secondary outcome.[99] Intervention components are summarized in KQ 1.

McKibbin et al.[105] conducted a fair-quality, randomized 6-month trial of a lifestyle intervention in older individuals (mean age=54.0) with schizophrenia and diabetes mellitus compared with modestly enhanced usual care as the control group (provision of three American Diabetes Association brochures and treatment by a primary care provider alone) (n=64). Consistent with diabetes, mean HbA1c levels were elevated at baseline (HbA1c=7.4 in the intervention group, 6.7 in the usual care group). Though the intervention was not fully described in the paper, elements of it were tailored to the SMI population, including having the intervention delivered by mental health professionals and delivered to groups of individuals who all had a diagnosis of schizophrenia. Though a completers analysis showed that mean HbA1c decreased in the intervention group to 6.9 and increased in the usual care group to 6.8, between-group differences were not significant (p=0.44). There were no differences in overall rates of study discontinuation. Specific reasons for discontinuation were reported for 7 of the 64 participants who did not complete the study. Of these, three would be considered serious adverse effects (inpatient hospitalization, n=2; death prior to study commencement, n=1; psychiatric decompensation, n=1). Based on mean Positive and Negative Syndrome Scale (PANSS) scores, there was no significant worsening of psychiatric symptoms among the study groups.

Gillhoff et al.[99] conducted a fair-quality randomized 5-month trial of a multicondition lifestyle intervention in individuals with bipolar disorder compared with a waitlist control group (n=50). The intervention was tailored to the SMI population in that the lifestyle and nutrition components (but not the fitness component) were delivered by mental health professionals. Additionally, the lifestyle component provided information about bipolar disorder. The total population mean baseline HbA1c was 5.5, with negligible between-group differences. Mean HbA1c changed minimally (0.1 or less) in the two groups at study completion and at 6-month followup, with a nonsignificant time by intervention term in a multivariate analysis (p-value not reported). Discontinuation due to adverse events and serious adverse events were not reported. Measures of psychiatric symptoms worsening were not reported.

Effect of Peer or Family Support Interventions on Diabetes Control
We identified no eligible studies for this category of intervention for KQ 2.

Effect of Pharmacological Treatments on Diabetes Control

Ramelteon
Only one study assessed the effects of a psychotropic agent on HbA1c.[92] In this fair-quality study, individuals with schizophrenia (n=20) were randomized to an 8-week trial of the MT1 and MT2 melatonin-selective antagonist ramelteon compared with placebo control. Mean HbA1c changed negligibly at 8 weeks, with no significant between-group difference in mean change at study end between ramelteon and placebo control (5.74 to 5.82 vs. 5.45 to 5.45, baseline to followup, p=0.61). Five participants (two in the ramelteon group and two in the placebo group) out of the 25 initially randomized withdrew consent before the Week 4 assessment. Reasons for discontinuation were not reported. No serious adverse effects were reported.

Metformin
Two studies evaluated interventions utilizing metformin, one with the primary target of metabolic control,[116] including glycemic control, and one with the primary target of obesity prevention[101] with glycemic control measured as a secondary outcome.

Carrizo et al.[116] conducted a fair-quality 14-week trial (61 participants) of extended release metformin in nondiabetic individuals receiving clozapine (94% with a diagnosis of schizophrenia) compared with placebo alone. The total population mean baseline HbA1c was 5.4, with negligible between-group differences. Mean HbA1c was increased modestly in both groups (+0.13 for metformin, +0.23 for placebo), though significantly less so in the metformin group (p=0.04). All 30 participants in the placebo group completed the study. No participant discontinued the study due to adverse effects, and no serious adverse effects were reported.

Hoffmann et al.[101] conducted a poor-quality 22-week trial of two treatment algorithms that included both metformin and amantadine added to olanzapine compared with olanzapine alone in nondiabetic individuals with schizophrenia or schizoaffective disorder for prevention of weight gain (199 participants). Baseline HcA1c values were not reported. Treatment algorithm A consisted of 200 mg amantadine with possible switches to 1000 to 1500 mg metformin and then switches to 100 to 400 mg zonisamide. Treatment algorithm B was 1000 to 1500 mg metformin, with possible switches to 200 mg amantadine and then switches to 100 to 400 mg zonisamide. A combined-treatment group of both algorithm A and algorithm B did not differ significantly from the olanzapine-only group at 22-week followup for HbA1c (results not reported, p=0.278). Mean change in HbA1c for the algorithm A arm was negligibly higher (+0.01) at followup than in the olanzapine-only group (p=0.976). However, patients treated with algorithm B (beginning with metformin, with possible switches to amantadine, and then to zonisamide) demonstrated a statistically significant (-0.03 vs. +0.09, p=0.049) improvement in mean changes compared with the olanzapine-only group in HbA1c values at followup, though the magnitude of the effect was small. In total, 14 participants discontinued the study due to adverse effects (8 in algorithm A group, 4 in algorithm B group, and 2 in olanzapine-only group); only three of these, all in algorithm A groups, were considered serious adverse effects. Ten participants continued the study despite serious adverse effects (1 in algorithm A group, 4 in algorithm B group, and 5 in olanzapine-only group). There was no significant worsening of psychiatric symptoms among the study groups for Brief Psychiatric Rating Scale and Clinical Global Impression-Severity (CGI-S) scores.

Effect of Antipsychotic-Switching Interventions on Diabetes Control

Two studies evaluated antipsychotic-switching strategies.[95,102] The primary outcome for these studies was weight management, with glycemic control measured as a secondary outcome. Patients in both studies began on olanzapine, and the control condition consisted of staying on olanzapine. The intervention involved switching to either quetiapine[95] or orally disintegrating olanzapine.[102] Neither study reported significant changes in HbA1c. Details are reported below. A third study, described in KQ 4, evaluated switching to aripiprazole as part of a multicomponent intervention. This study found no effect on HbA1c.

Deberdt et al.[95] conducted a fair-quality 24-week trial of switching from olanzapine (baseline dose of 7.5 to 20 mg/day) to quetiapine (300 to 800 mg/day) in overweight or obese individuals with schizophrenia or schizoaffective disorder compared with staying on olanzapine (n=133). The total population mean baseline HbA1c was 5.9. Final mean modal daily doses for patients switching to quetiapine (n=68) and staying on olanzapine (n=65) were 16.9 mg and 439.7 mg, respectively. Patients who switched to quetiapine did not have significantly different changes in their HbA1c levels than those who remained on olanzapine (+0.07 and -0.03, p=0.318) in the last-outcome-carried-forward analysis. Significantly more patients in the olanzapine group completed 24 weeks of treatment than in the quetiapine group (70.3% vs. 43.1%, p=0.002).

Adverse effects leading to study discontinuation were classified as psychiatric adverse events and nonpsychiatric adverse events. Discontinuations due to psychiatric adverse events were more frequent in the quetiapine group than the olanzapine group (p=0.031). No significant differences were demonstrated for discontinuations due to nonpsychiatric adverse events or due to lack of efficacy, though a significant difference favoring olanzapine was demonstrated for the combination of discontinuations due to psychiatric adverse events or lack of efficacy. There were no significant differences in hospitalization rates (7.69% in the quetiapine group vs. 1.47% in the olanzapine group, p-value not reported). No other serious adverse events were reported. Based on mean PANSS scores, neither study arm demonstrated worsening of psychiatric symptoms.

Karagianis et al.[102] conducted a good-quality 16-week trial of switching from standard olanzapine tablets to orally disintegrating olanzapine in individuals with schizophrenia, schizoaffective disorder, bipolar disorder, or another related psychotic disorder who had gained significant weight (defined as 5 kg or more or an increase of 1 kg/m^2 in BMI) while on standard olanzapine tablets for 4 to 52 weeks compared with remaining on standard olanzapine tablets (n=149). The total population mean baseline HbA1c was 5.5, with negligible between-group differences. The final mean daily dose in the standard olanzapine tablets group (n=65) was 14.90 mg. Final mean daily dose in the orally disintegrating olanzapine group (n=84) was 14.33 mg. Patients who switched to orally disintegrating olanzapine did not have significantly different changes in their HbA1c levels from those who remained on olanzapine (+0.0 and +0.0, p=0.83). Results for health-related quality of life as measured by the Subjective Well-being Under Neuroleptics Scale showed no significant change from baseline to followup between groups (p=0.16). Two patients in each group discontinued treatment due to adverse effects. Two patients in the orally disintegrating olanzapine group experienced serious adverse effects, with one being hospitalized for dizziness and one attempting suicide. There was no significant worsening of psychiatric symptoms between groups as measured by the CGI-S scale.

Summary of Key Question 2

Only one of the seven studies relevant to KQ 2 tested an intervention specifically intended to improve glucose control in individuals with diabetes and SMI.[105] Of the other six studies, two had HbA1c as among the primary outcomes,[92,116] and four focused more specifically on weight, with HbA1c measured as a secondary outcome.[95,99,101,102] Overall, just two of the trials found significant advantages for the intervention in controlling HbA1c, with both of these studies involving the use of metformin. Carrizo et al.[116] demonstrated that metformin in nondiabetic individuals receiving clozapine led to significantly less increase in HbA1c during the 14-week study. Hoffmann et al.[101] showed that a treatment algorithm, beginning with metformin and possible switches to amantadine and then to zonisamide, demonstrated a statistically significant improvement in mean changes in HbA1c when added to olanzapine treatment in nondiabetic individuals compared with those receiving only olanzapine over 22 weeks. In both of these instances, mean advantages for the interventions were modest (-0.10 to -0.12). Behavioral interventions,[99,105] antipsychotic switching,[95,102] and the psychotropic drug ramelteon[92] resulted in no significant differences in HbA1c control in individuals with SMI. Outcomes regarding weight and lipids are summarized in KQ 1 and KQ 3, respectively. In brief, health-related quality of life and serious adverse events were inconsistently reported in the seven trials. Health-related quality of life was reported in only one of the trials with no significant effect demonstrated. No trials reported on mortality.

Key Question 3. Effectiveness of Dyslipidemia-Management Interventions

KQ 3: What is the effectiveness of dyslipidemia-management behavioral interventions (e.g., behavioral counseling, health education), peer or family support interventions, pharmacological treatments (e.g., statins), antipsychotic medication–switching to an antipsychotic with a low or neutral impact on lipid levels, or their combination on lipid-level control and related physical health outcomes (e.g., health-related quality of life, mortality) when compared with each other or with usual care (or other control) among adults with SMI who have dyslipidemia or are taking antipsychotics?

Key Points

- Lipid levels have not been a primary target for interventions studied in individuals with SMI. While 15 RCTs reported lipid levels as a secondary outcome (the studies included in this section), no studies evaluated an intervention specifically designed to target lipid levels in individuals with SMI who have or are at risk for dyslipidemia. Hence, the strength of evidence for each intervention examined in KQ 3 is insufficient.
- Interventions known to be effective for managing dyslipidemia, such as medications (e.g., HMG-CoA reductase inhibitors) or dietary interventions, have not been studied in SMI populations. It seems that such interventions should be considered for clinical use, but direct evidence in SMI populations is lacking.
- Behavioral interventions were found in a meta-analysis to have no advantage over usual care for managing low-density lipoprotein (LDL) levels, but this analysis consisted of three small, 3- to 12-month studies aimed primarily at either weight or diabetes management.
- Small improvements in lipids were seen in one study of ramelteon, one study of topiramate, and one study that used a sequenced medication algorithm of amantadine, metformin, and zonisamide.
- Lipid levels improved modestly in two studies of aripiprazole—one that added aripiprazole to chronic clozapine and one that switched patients from olanzapine to aripiprazole. Switching from oral to injectable olanzapine increased LDL cholesterol.

Detailed Synthesis

We identified no articles reporting on trials in which the intervention was designed to target lipid levels. Specifically, no study evaluated HMG-CoA reductase inhibitors (statins), niacin, fibrates, or low-fat diets. However, 15 of the eligible studies, involving 2322 patients, reported on total cholesterol (n=12) or LDL cholesterol (n=14) as a secondary outcome.[89,91,92,95,98-102,105,106,108,114,115,119] All of these trials were published from 2005 forward, with reported recruitment dates spanning from 2001 to 2010. The primary outcomes of interest were weight (n=12), glucose control (n=1), and all-purpose metabolic effects (n=2). Of the 15 trials that reported on lipid levels, all 15 were included in KQ 1 (weight), 7 were included in KQ 2 (glucose control), and none were included in KQ 4 (multicondition interventions). Detailed analyses of the outcomes for weight control (KQ 1) and glucose control (KQ 2) are presented in other sections of the Results chapter. The experimental intervention was psychotropic medication in three trials, antipsychotic switching in four trials, behavioral interventions in three trials, neurological agents in three trials, an antihistamine in one trial, and a neurological agent or a biguanide in one trial (this trial was the only one with three arms instead of two).

Common inclusion criteria were a diagnosis of schizophrenia (n=12), taking an antipsychotic medication (n=10), and being overweight or obese (n=7). Common exclusion criteria were active substance abuse (n=7), being pregnant or breastfeeding (n=8), being on non-study approved medication (n=8), and having a chronic medical condition (n=12). The number of participants randomized ranged from 21 to 1065, and the number who completed studies ranged from 18 to 677.

Trials received funding from private industries (n=13) and government (n=4). Five of the 15 studies were conducted in multiple countries, with patients coming from the United States in 8 studies, Europe in 5 studies, Asia in 2 studies, South America in 1 study, and Africa in 1 study. Six studies were conducted at a single study site, and 4 studies contained 19 or more study sites. One study contained 112 study centers across 26 countries.[108] This study contained 44 percent of the overall number of patients across the 15 studies, with samples from the 6 largest studies[95,98,101,102,106,108] accounting for 81 percent of the total sample size for KQ 3.

Study Characteristics

Table 9 shows the study characteristics for KQ 3. The majority of patients were male, white, and middle-aged. The vast majority were classified as having schizophrenia or schizoaffective disorder (92%), with 6 percent having bipolar disorder and less than 2 percent classified as having serious mental illness not further specified. None of the studies reported on whether patients were diagnosed with hyperlipidemia. Average baseline total cholesterol and LDL levels for most studies were in a clinically acceptable range. Patients in the large majority of studies were reported as taking a second-generation antipsychotic medication. Studies were conducted primarily in outpatient mental health settings and most commonly examined medication compared with placebo. Nine studies lasted 2 to 4 months, four studies lasted 5 to 6 months, and two studies lasted 11 to 12 months. Most studies were rated fair quality, with common reasons for reduced study quality being insufficient details provided about the study, inadequate blinding, and conducting analyses only on treatment completers. There was a relatively even split between trials that were characterized as efficacy studies and those characterized as a mixed efficacy–effectiveness.

Table 9. Study characteristics for KQ 3: Dyslipidemia-management interventions

Characteristic	Details
Studies: N (patients)[a]	15 studies (2322 patients)
Mean age of sample: Median (range)	39.0 (31.1 to 54.0)

Sex: N patients (%)
  Female
  Male
  NR
	810 patients (35%)
	1379 patients (59%)
	133 patients (6%)

Race: N patients (%)
  White
  Nonwhite
  NR
	1408 patients (61%)
	603 patients (26%)
	299 patients (13%)

Mean lipid levels: Median (range)
  Total cholesterol
  LDL
	198 mg/dl (133 mg/dl to 212 mg/dl)
	120 mg/dl (72 mg/dl to 138 mg/dl)

Setting: N studies (%)
  Mental health outpatient
  Outpatient setting not otherwise specified
  Community
  NR
	9 studies (60%)
	2 studies (13%)
	1 study (7%)
	3 studies (20%)

Study quality: N studies (%)[b]
  Good
  Fair
  Poor
	4 studies (27%)
	8 studies (53%)
	3 studies (20%)

Efficacy–effectiveness rating: N studies (%)
  Efficacy (0–2)
  Mixed (3–5)
  Effectiveness (6–7)
	8 studies (53%)
	7 studies (47%)
	0 studies (0%)

Comparisons: N studies (patients)
  Drug vs. placebo/control
  Behavioral vs. control
  Antipsychotic switching vs. antipsychotic stay
  Drug vs. drug vs. placebo control
	7 studies (447 patients)
	3 studies (156 patients)
	4 studies (1520 patients)
	1 study (199 patients)

LDL = low-density lipoprotein; N = number; NR = not reported

[a]The number of patients with demographic data reported is fewer than the number randomized.

[b]Quality ratings in the table are reported on the basis of how studies were conducted in relation to physical health outcomes. Ratings were also applied on the basis of psychiatric outcomes. Quality ratings did not differ for any studies on the basis of physical versus psychiatric outcomes.

Meta-Analysis and Qualitative Review

There was a sufficient number of studies with cohesive intervention strategies to conduct a meta-analysis only for the effect of behavioral interventions on lipid levels. Results for the other effects are summarized qualitatively.

Effect of Behavioral Interventions on Lipid Control

Figure 9 shows the forest plot of the meta-analysis examining the effect of behavioral interventions on LDL levels, which included two fair-quality studies[99,105] and one poor-quality study[114] (156 patients). Two of the behavioral interventions focused on weight management, and one focused on diabetes management. All interventions included components that focused on physical activity and exercise as well as on diet and nutrition. Interventions were adapted for SMI populations by simplifying content to focus on key points (e.g., introducing only one or two topics per session) and by employing concrete behavioral change strategies (e.g., food diaries, pedometers). The number of planned contacts ranged from 7 to 24 sessions, and duration of followup ranged from 3 to 12 months. Control conditions consisted of waitlist, no intervention, and usual care plus information (see Table 7 in KQ 1 section for details). These control group conditions were combined in the meta-analysis, as participants in waitlist and no intervention conditions were allowed to continue receiving usual care.

Figure 9. Forest plot of meta-analysis of effect of behavioral interventions on LDL levels

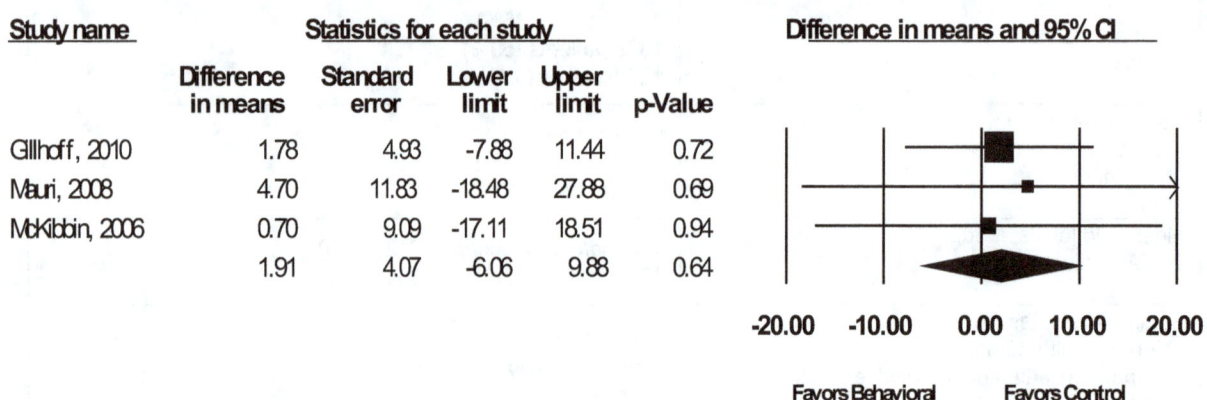

Study name	Statistics for each study					Difference in means and 95% CI
	Difference in means	Standard error	Lower limit	Upper limit	p-Value	
Gillhoff, 2010	1.78	4.93	-7.88	11.44	0.72	
Mauri, 2008	4.70	11.83	-18.48	27.88	0.69	
McKibbin, 2006	0.70	9.09	-17.11	18.51	0.94	
	1.91	4.07	-6.06	9.88	0.64	

CI = confidence interval; LDL = low-density lipoprotein

The analysis revealed no statistically significant difference in efficacy between behavioral interventions and control for managing LDL levels (mean difference, 1.91 mg/dl; 95% CI, -6.06 to 9.88), with no evidence of heterogeneity (Cochran Q=0.07, df=2, p=0.96; I^2=0%). Again, because formal statistical techniques for publication bias are not effective with small numbers of studies, we did not conduct analyses for publication bias. Only one of the three studies on behavioral interventions reported on adverse effects as defined in our study protocol,[114] which reported that no drug-related severe adverse effects were observed. None of the studies reported on health-related quality of life.

Only two of the behavioral intervention studies reported on total cholesterol. In a 5-month multimodal lifestyle intervention that consisted of 11 group sessions and weekly fitness training for bipolar disorder patients (n=50), no significant differences were found between those in the lifestyle intervention group and those in a waiting control group.[99] In a 3-month psychoeducational program for weight control in patients who experienced weight gain on olanzapine (n=33), there were no significant differences in total cholesterol between those in the psychoeducational program and those receiving no intervention.[114]

Effect of Peer or Family Support Interventions on Lipid Control
We identified no eligible studies for this category of intervention for KQ 3.

Effect of Pharmacological Treatments on Lipid Control

Psychotropic Agents
A total of one good-quality[98] and two fair-quality[91,92] studies examined the effect of psychotropic medications on lipids (321 patients). Two of these studies recorded data on total cholesterol and all three studies on LDL. Study medications were ramelteon, aripiprazole, and atomoxetine, and the comparator in each study was placebo. The study durations ranged from 2 to 6 months.

Although ramelteon, aripiprazole, and atomoxetine all can be classified as psychotropic medications, we did not conduct a meta-analysis on the studies using these medications because their mechanisms of action vary substantially. Indeed, when examined qualitatively, results were mixed. The 24-week study of overweight schizophrenia patients (n=37) taking olanzapine or clozapine who were randomized to atomoxetine or placebo did not measure total cholesterol levels and found no difference between groups on change in LDL levels.[91] However, two of the studies did find significant change between groups. The small 8-week pilot trial on ramelteon (n=25) found that stable outpatients with schizophrenia were significantly more likely to experience a decrease in total cholesterol (-9.79 mg/dl loss vs. 3.84 mg/dl gain, p=.03) when taking ramelteon than placebo.[92] Change in LDL levels displayed the same pattern, but group differences were not significant in this small study. Groups did not significantly differ on changes in psychiatric symptoms over the course of this study. In a 16-week trial of aripiprazole versus placebo among 207 schizophrenia patients who had experienced weight gain while taking clozapine,[98] those in the aripiprazole group had greater percentage reductions in their total cholesterol levels (-6.9% vs. -1.2%, p=.002) and LDL levels (-10.3% vs. 0.0%, p=.003). Psychiatric symptoms improved more in the aripiprazole group over the course of this study (p=.037).

Of the three studies examining the effect on lipid levels of adding medication, none found significant changes between groups on psychiatric symptoms, and only one reported on health-related quality of life or on serious adverse effects as defined by the study protocol.[98] This study found no significant differences between patients taking aripiprazole as an adjunctive medication to clozapine and patients taking placebo and clozapine on a measure of subjective well-being, but the study did find 0 out of 99 patients in the placebo group and 10 out of 108 patients in the aripiprazole group to experience a serious adverse effect.

Neurological Agents

The effect of neurological agents on lipids was examined in one good-quality,[115] one fair-quality,[119] and two poor-quality[100,101] trials. Three of these studies employed a two-arm design (135 patients),[100,115,119] and one study used a three-arm design (199 patients).[101] In all two-arm studies, the control condition was placebo. Study medications were amantadine, topiramate, and zonisamide (the three-arm study also involved metformin), and study durations ranged from 3 to 5 months. We were unable to complete meta-analysis on these studies due to heterogeneous study designs and unreported lipid outcome data (one study[100] stated only that results for lipids were not significant).

Results were mixed in the three two-arm studies that examined neurological agents compared with placebo. A 12-week study of amantadine versus placebo among 21 patients who had gained at least 5 pounds on olanzapine found no differences between groups on total cholesterol or LDL levels.[100] In a 12-week study of 72 first-episode schizophrenia patients randomized to either olanzapine plus topiramate or olanzapine plus placebo,[119] patients taking topiramate were significantly less likely than those in the placebo group to experience a rise in LDL levels (0.34 mg% rise vs. 10.53 mg% rise, p=.009). Finally, a 16-week study of zonisamide versus placebo in 42 patients beginning olanzapine for bipolar disorder or schizophrenia found no significant differences between groups on total cholesterol or LDL levels.[115] None of these three studies reported on health-related quality of life or serious adverse effects.

The three-arm, 22-week study[101] examined two different medication treatment-switching algorithms for prevention of weight gain compared with no medication in 199 patients with schizophrenia or schizoaffective disorder who were all taking olanzapine. The algorithms using amantadine, metformin, and zonisamide were significantly more effective at preventing increases in total cholesterol than olanzapine treatment alone (0.18 mg/dl gain and -1.44 mg/dl loss on algorithms vs. 6.49 mg/dl gain on olanzapine alone). The algorithms had a less pronounced and nonsignificant effect for LDL. Health-related quality of life was not measured. Thirteen patients experienced a serious adverse effect, and a total of 14 patients discontinued the study due to a serious or nonserious adverse effect (group differences not tested).

Nizatidine

A 12-week, good-quality study that examined the efficacy of nizatidine versus placebo for weight management in 54 patients with schizophrenia taking olanzapine found no statistically significant differences between groups with respect to the intervention's effect on lipid levels.[89] The study did not measure health-related quality of life. There was no significant difference between groups with respect to adverse effects, with one patient in the nizatidine group and two patients in the placebo group discontinuing due to an adverse effect.

Effect of Antipsychotic-Switching Interventions on Lipid Control

There was a total of one good-quality[102] and three fair-quality[95,106,108] studies (1376 patients) that examined the effect of switching antipsychotic medications on lipids. Patients in all studies began on olanzapine, and in all studies the control condition consisted of staying on olanzapine. The intervention in two studies involved switching to a different form of olanzapine (an orally disintegrating tablet or a long-acting injection) and in the other two studies involved switching to a different antipsychotic medication (quetiapine or aripiprazole). Study durations ranged from 4 to 6 months. Meta-analysis was not completed on these four studies due to the heterogeneity of switching strategies.

There were mixed results in the two studies that examined switching to a different form of olanzapine.[102,108] In the 16-week trial of 149 patients with SMI that involved switching from standard olanzapine tablets to orally disintegrating olanzapine tablets,[102] there was no difference between groups with respect to lipid levels. This study found no difference between groups on a measure of subjective well-being. Serious adverse effects were experienced by two patients in the orally disintegrating olanzapine group and none in the standard olanzapine tablet group.

In the 24-week trial of 921 patients with schizophrenia that involved switching from oral olanzapine to a long-acting injection of olanzapine,[108] patients continuing oral olanzapine experienced a significantly greater decrease in LDL levels than did patients in the long-acting injection group (-6.4 mg/dl loss vs. -1.5 mg/dl loss, p=.039). The groups did not differ on total cholesterol. This study did not measure health-related quality of life. Serious adverse effects were reported in 12 patients, and 57 patients discontinued due to adverse effects, but the authors report that there was no statistically significant difference between groups for adverse effects.

The studies that examined switching from olanzapine to a different antipsychotic medication[95,106] also had mixed results. In the 24-week study of 133 overweight patients with schizophrenia that examined switching from olanzapine to quetiapine,[95] those who switched to quetiapine did not have significantly different changes in their total cholesterol or LDL levels than those who remained on olanzapine. This study did not report on health-related quality of life or serious adverse effects as defined by study protocol. While the study found no difference between groups on treatment-emergent adverse events, discontinuation was significantly higher in the quetiapine group (56.9% discontinued vs. 29.4%, p=.002). In the 16-week trial of 173 patients with schizophrenia who either stayed on olanzapine or switched to aripiprazole,[106] those who switched to aripiprazole had a significantly greater percentage decrease in total cholesterol

(-9.5% vs. -3.3%, p=.005) and a nonsignificantly greater percentage decrease in LDL (-11.2% vs. -4.7%, p=.072). This study did not report on health-related quality of life but did find that six aripiprazole-treated patients experienced a serious adverse effect and seven discontinued, compared with nine olanzapine-treated patients who experienced a serious adverse effect and eight who discontinued.

Summary of Key Question 3

None of the 15 studies in KQ 3 contained an intervention specifically intended to target lipid levels. Instead, the primary outcomes of interest were weight in 12 of the studies, glucose control in 1 study, and all-purpose metabolic effects in 2 studies. Total cholesterol was measured in 12 studies and LDL in 14 studies. Overall, 6 of the 15 trials found significant changes between study groups on lipid levels. The interventions in these studies included ramelteon,[92] topiramate,[119] medication treatment algorithms,[101] and aripiprazole.[98,106] In all instances, intervention effects resulted in a 5-percent or less difference in lipid values compared with control (placebo or stay on original medication). Also, one study testing a long-acting injection of olanzapine found that participants receiving the injection were less likely than those remaining on oral olanzapine to experience a decrease in LDL.[108] Since all studies were evaluating lipids as a secondary outcome and are summarized in KQ 1, the details regarding other health outcomes are summarized in that section. In brief, health-related quality of life and serious adverse effects were infrequently reported in the 15 trials. Health-related quality of life was reported in only 2 of the 15 trials. Serious adverse effects were reported in four studies, and adverse effects leading to treatment discontinuation were reported in seven studies.

Key Question 4. Effectiveness of Multicondition Lifestyle Interventions

KQ 4: What is the effectiveness of multicondition lifestyle interventions (e.g., combinations of smoking cessation, physical activity, and nutrition counseling with or without medication management) on cardiovascular risk factors and related physical health outcomes (e.g., health-related quality of life, mortality) among adults with SMI who have cardiovascular disease, elevated cardiovascular risk (e.g., hypertension), or are taking antipsychotics?

Key Points

- Only three studies evaluated lifestyle interventions. Lifestyle interventions consisted primarily of dietary and exercise components. One study offered additional provisions such as heart rate monitors and financial subsidies to support the exercise component.
- One study reported small to moderate beneficial effects on body mass index (BMI), weight, and cholesterol:
  - This good-quality study showed benefit in switching from olanzapine, quetiapine, or risperidone to aripiprazole in the context of a manualized, behaviorally oriented diet and exercise program.

45

- The effects of the behavioral component of the lifestyle intervention in this study are unknown, since both the intervention and comparison arm received the behavioral component.
- Two studies reported significant benefits of multicondition lifestyle interventions for self-reported health-related quality of life.
- Studies included in KQ 4 varied substantially on methodological rigor and quality variables.
- Overall, the evidence is insufficient to estimate the effects of multicondition lifestyle interventions.

Detailed Synthesis

Studies relevant to KQ 4 evaluated multicondition lifestyle interventions (e.g., combinations of behavioral and medication management, broadly conceived behavioral interventions) for more than one CVD risk factor (e.g., metabolic syndrome) or health condition. We identified 3 studies involving 286 patients that assessed the effects of lifestyle interventions on CVD risk factors and related physical health outcomes among adults with SMI.[120-122] Two of these studies evaluated broadly conceived behavioral interventions, and one evaluated the combination of antipsychotic switching in combination with a behavioral intervention. No study addressed multiple conditions associated with CVD risk such as obesity, diabetes mellitus, and hypertension.

Study Characteristics

Table 10 shows the study characteristics for KQ 4. The diagnostic samples identified by these studies included schizophrenia-only[120] and SMI (i.e., psychotic and mood disorders).[121,122] Two studies were conducted in the United States[120,122] and one in Europe.[121] One study[120] was conducted in several clinical research centers, while one[121] was conducted in supported housing facilities. The third study[122] reported that recruitment was conducted at a large mental health facility's inpatient and outpatient programs and surrounding community treatment centers, but the location of intervention delivery was unclear. Compared with studies included in the other KQs, these studies had less restrictive exclusion criteria. Thus, participants could have been included who had other comorbid physical conditions. The study by Stroup et al.[120] was rated as a mixed efficacy–effectiveness study of good quality, Forsberg et al.[121] as a mixed efficacy–effectiveness study of fair quality, and Skrinar et al.[122] as an efficacy study of fair quality.

Table 10. Study characteristics for KQ 4: Multicondition lifestyle interventions

Characteristic	Details
Studies: N studies (patients)[a]	3 studies (286 patients)
Mean age of sample: Median (range)	41.0 (41.0 to 37.8)

Sex: N patients (%)
  Female
  Male
  NR
	114 patients (40%)
	172 patients (60%)
	0 patients (0%)

Race: N patients (%)
  White
  Nonwhite
  NR
	123 patients (43%)
	90 patients (31%)
	73 patients (26%)

Setting: N studies (%)[b]
  Mental health
  General medical
  Community
  Integrated mental health-medical
	2 studies (67%)
	0 studies (0%)
	2 studies (67%)
	0 studies (0%)

Study quality: N studies (%)
  Good
  Fair
  Poor
	1 study (33%)
	2 studies (67%)
	0 studies (0%)

Efficacy–effectiveness rating: N studies (%)
  Efficacy (0–2)
  Mixed (3–5)
  Effectiveness (6–7)
	1 study (33%)
	2 studies (66%)
	0 studies (0%)

Comparisons: N studies (patients)
  Drug + behavioral vs. drug
  Lifestyle intervention vs. control
	1 study (215 patients)
	2 studies (71 patients)

Mean BMI (study range)	3 studies (21.55 to 35)
Mean HbA1c% (study range)	2 studies (4.16 to 6.0)
Mean systolic blood pressure	1 study (133.9)
Mean total cholesterol	1 study (217)
Mean non-HDL cholesterol	1 study (173)
Current smoker: N studies; N patients (%) NR	1 study; 19 of 41 patients (46%) 2 studies; 286 patients
Metabolic syndrome: N patients (%) NR	1 study; 21 of 41 patients (51%) 2 studies; 286 patients

BMI = body mass index; HbA1c = hemoglobin A1c; HDL = high-density lipoprotein; N = number; NR = not reported
[a]The number of patients with demographic data reported is fewer than the number randomized.
[b]Stroup et al.[120] selected participants from both mental health and community settings.

Qualitative Review

The three studies included in KQ 4 are described below qualitatively due to the variability in interventions and outcomes.

Effect of Multicondition Lifestyle Interventions on Cardiovascular Risk Factors

In a fair-quality mixed efficacy–effectiveness study by Forsberg et al.,[121] 46 participants were randomized to receive either a health intervention program or a non–health-related control program for 12 months. Demographic and outcome data were reported for the 41 participants who completed the study. Importantly, participants were recruited from supported housing facilities. The health intervention program, aimed at improving physical health, provided group dietary education, physical activity sessions, provision of a heart rate monitor, and a 50-percent financial subsidy that supported entrance at sports centers and equipment rental. Group sessions were 2 hours in duration and were held twice weekly for the entire 12-month study. The control group attended art classes held once weekly for 2 hours.

At baseline, rates of schizophrenia (intervention=17, control=6) and metabolic syndrome (intervention=16, control=5) were significantly higher in the resident intervention group compared with the resident control group. At followup, no significant differences between the active and control groups were reported for BMI, weight in kilograms, HbA1c percentage, systolic blood pressure, diastolic blood pressure, smoking cessation, or a composite CVD risk score at 13.5 months. There was a significant decrease in the number of individuals diagnosed with metabolic syndrome in the intervention group (from 13 to 10), while there was a nonsignificant increase in the number of individuals diagnosed with metabolic syndrome in the control group (from 4 to 6); however, these changes did not differ significantly between the intervention and control groups. This was true also for systolic blood pressure, which demonstrated a significant decrease from baseline to followup in the intervention group (from 139.0 to 124.9), but no between-group difference was observed. After the authors controlled for sex and age, a significant reduction in triglycerides was observed for participants over 40 years of age in both groups; between-group change was nonsignificant. A performance-based measure of physical functioning, the incremental shuttle walk test, was not affected by the intervention. Adverse effects were not reported. Quality issues included low attendance at group sessions, inability of the researchers to control whether participants in the comparison condition engaged in exercise or dieting while enrolled, no intent-to-treat analysis, and absence of a description of the antipsychotic medication status of study participants.

In a fair-quality efficacy study by Skrinar et al.,[122] 30 individuals with SMI were randomized to a healthy lifestyle group or to a waitlist control group for 12 weeks; outcome data were reported for the 20 participants who completed the study. Participants in this study were recruited from inpatient and outpatient units and from a community treatment facility. The healthy lifestyle intervention consisted of four exercise sessions each week and weekly health seminars covering a broad range of topics (e.g., healthy eating, weight management, stress relief) and intended to target weight gain and physical fitness. Participants in the control group were offered the exercise intervention following the initial 12-week study period and were informed that it was not necessary to limit physical activity. Both the lifestyle and control groups kept detailed logs of any exercise sessions.

There were no significant differences between groups at 12 weeks for BMI, weight, total cholesterol, glucose, or psychiatric symptom severity (as measured by the Symptom Checklist-90 score). Participants in the intervention group showed significantly greater increases in their subjective rating of general health as measured by the General Health factor of the SF-36 scale (intervention group mean difference, 13.64 vs. control group, -4.09, p=.01). Self-reported physical health and role limitations due to physical health also improved more in the intervention group, but the differences were not statistically significant. Adverse effects were not reported. Quality issues included low adherence rate (63%), small sample size, and lack of an intent-to-treat analysis. Study authors noted specific barriers to participation in the intervention (e.g., transportation, financial issues), which contributed to the low adherence rate—highlighting a common challenge of exercise interventions in the SMI population. They emphasized the positive impact of the intervention on perceived health-related well-being despite the lack of significant behavioral or metabolic changes.

In contrast to the other two studies, the third study by Stroup et al.[120] was a large (n=215), good-quality, mixed efficacy–effectiveness trial (Comparison of Antipsychotics for Metabolic Problems) carried out between January 2007 and March 2010. This study examined the impact of switching from the antipsychotics olanzapine, quetiapine, or risperidone to aripiprazole (flexible dose) on weight and metabolic variables. All participants in the study took part in a manualized, behaviorally oriented diet and exercise program (once weekly visits for the first month, followed by once monthly visits thereafter) that was based on previous group protocols used with SMI populations.[82,93] After the first 4 weeks, study personnel contacted participants with a telephone call to reinforce the behavioral treatment lessons between each of the monthly visits. Laboratory assessments were conducted every 4 weeks. The trial was carried out at 27 clinical research centers affiliated with the Schizophrenia Trials Network in the United States and was 24 weeks in duration. Participants were required to have a BMI greater than or equal to 27 and a non-HDL cholesterol greater than or equal to 130 mg/dl in order to be study eligible. The intervention arm of this study was intended to target metabolic risk factors for cardiovascular disease and included multiple outcomes of interest.

Overall, the results of this study supported switching to aripiprazole combined with a behavioral health-management program as a useful method for managing weight gain and metabolic problems in individuals with SMI and antipsychotic-related weight gain. Significant group effects were observed for BMI (mean difference, -1.1; p<.01), weight (mean difference, -2.9 kg; p<.01), total cholesterol (mean difference, -8.8 mg/dl; p=.02), and non-HDL cholesterol (mean difference, -9.4 mg/dl; p=.01). Stroup et al.[120] also reported significant intervention effects for health-related quality of life as indicated by the 12-Item Short-Form Health Survey for physical health (mean difference, 3.7; p<.02) and the Impact of Weight on Quality of Life–Lite Questionnaire (mean difference, -9.5; p<.01), with an advantage on both of these measures for patients who switched to aripiprazole. Serious adverse effects occurred in 16.8 percent of the group who switched to aripiprazole and 13.1 percent of those remaining on their current antipsychotic treatment (p-value not reported). There were no significant group effects for psychiatric symptoms as measured by the CGI-S assessment.

The biggest limitation of this study was differential attrition, with 47.7 percent of participants who switched medication discontinuing the study for any reason compared with 27.4 percent of those who did not switch. The authors speculated that this was due to clinician detection of clinical worsening in the switch group, which was confirmed in a post-hoc analysis. This highlights the need for careful clinical monitoring following medication switching. Despite the high rate of attrition, we rated the study as good quality since the authors thoroughly examined and accounted for incomplete data, and the study rated high on many other aspects of quality (e.g., performance bias, detection bias). Unlike the other two studies included in KQ 4, this study detected significant differential effects on weight and metabolic variables between the study groups. Although this study is informative with regard to medication switching, it did not examine the specific effect of the behavioral intervention, which all participants received. Therefore, we cannot speculate on the impact of this aspect of the lifestyle intervention beyond the effects of the medication.

Summary of Key Question 4

Only three published studies met inclusion criteria for KQ 4. The small number of RCTs and narrow range of interventions preclude drawing strong conclusions about the efficacy or effectiveness of multicondition lifestyle interventions on CVD risk factors or physical health outcomes for adults with SMI. Because these studies were highly inclusive of participants and outcomes (containing any study that targeted more than one condition), the specific physical parameters targeted were broad or at times loosely defined.

The behavioral component of the identified studies focused only on exercise and nutrition. One study also provided heart rate monitors and financial subsidies to support the physical activity component. No studies added components such as medication adherence, smoking cessation, or skills training (e.g., meal planning) that would have constituted a more comprehensive behavioral intervention. Further, no studies evaluated lifestyle interventions in combination with medications for weight loss (e.g., orlistat) or metabolic risk factors such as HMG-CoA reductase inhibitors for hyperlipidemia. The most important signal from these studies is that switching to aripiprazole—in combination with a structured behavioral intervention—is a promising strategy for minimizing adverse metabolic consequences of second-generation antipsychotics. However, the tradeoff may be a higher rate of worsening psychiatric status for the individual with SMI. Multicondition interventions demonstrated some promise for affecting health-related quality of life, as indicated by the effects of two of the three included studies.

Discussion

Key Findings and Strength of Evidence

We identified 35 trials that tested a wide array of pharmacological and behavioral interventions to address one or more CVD risk factors in adults with SMI who have elevated risk for CVD. Given that CVD is the most prevalent cause of death in this population, this is a surprisingly small number of studies. Further, we identified no peer and family support interventions to address elevated CVD risk, nor did we find any interventions designed specifically to address lipids. No interventions targeted individuals with psychotic depression specifically. Outcomes reported were primarily metabolic outcomes such as glucose control or weight; effects on physical function and overall CVD risk (e.g., Framingham Risk Score) were reported infrequently, and all-cause mortality was not reported.

Table 11 presents a brief overview of key findings by intervention as well as the strength of evidence (SOE) by KQ for major outcomes. The drug classes in our review sometimes included drugs with diverse mechanisms of action. When results varied by drug, we assigned separate SOE. Publication bias was difficult to assess because only a few comparisons had sufficient studies for statistical analysis. For adverse effects, we considered discontinuation due to adverse effects and worsening of psychiatric status as the key outcomes when rating SOE. When the majority of studies reported only one of these outcomes, we considered the evidence for adverse effects incomplete and rated the limited evidence as indirect. In brief, evidence was insufficient for most intervention strategies, and there were too few studies to conduct quantitative synthesis for all outcomes of interest, except for weight.

Table 11. Overview of treatment effects and SOE by intervention and major outcomes[a]

Intervention	KQ 1: Weight	KQ 2: Diabetes (HbA1c)	KQ 3: Lipids[b]	Overall CVD Risk and Other Outcomes
Behavioral	Small benefit (-3.1 kg) Moderate SOE	Insufficient SOE	No important effect from weight control interventions Insufficient SOE	1 study assessed health-related quality of life and found no differences Only 2 studies reported discontinuation due to adverse effects Insufficient SOE
Peer or family support	No studies Insufficient SOE	No studies Insufficient SOE	No studies Insufficient SOE	No studies Insufficient SOE
Metformin	Small benefit (-4.1 kg) Low SOE	Insufficient SOE	No studies Insufficient SOE	Insufficient SOE for CVD risk
Topiramate, zonisamide	Small to moderate benefit (-5.1 kg) Low SOE	Insufficient SOE	Possible benefit with topiramate Insufficient SOE	Insufficient SOE for CVD risk

Table 11. Overview of treatment effects and SOE by intervention and major outcomes[a] (continued)

Intervention	KQ 1: Weight	KQ 2: Diabetes (HbA1c)	KQ 3: Lipids[b]	Overall CVD Risk and Other Outcomes
Antihistamine	No benefit Low SOE	Insufficient SOE	Single study did not suggest benefit Insufficient SOE	Insufficient SOE for CVD risk
Other medications	Insufficient SOE	Insufficient SOE	No study suggested possible benefit Insufficient SOE	Insufficient SOE for CVD risk
Antipsychotic switching or adjunctive use	Low SOE for small benefit (-2 to -3 kg) with switching to aripiprazole or adjunctive aripiprazole Insufficient SOE from single studies that found no effect with switching to quetiapine or parenteral olanzapine	Insufficient SOE	Possible benefit with adjunctive or switching to aripiprazole Low SOE	Insufficient SOE for CVD risk Low SOE for possible higher rate of mental health worsening with switching
Multicomponent lifestyle	Insufficient SOE	Insufficient SOE	Insufficient SOE	2 studies suggested benefit for health-related quality of life 1 study reported no benefit on CVD risk score Insufficient SOE

CVD = cardiovascular disease; HbA1c = hemoglobin A1c; KQ = Key Question; SOE = strength of evidence
[a]Shaded cells highlight SOE ratings that are above insufficient.
[b]No studies of lipid-focused interventions.

Key Question 1: Weight Control

The largest number of studies (32 of 35) addressed weight control. We found moderate SOE that behavioral interventions are associated with small decreases in weight (about 3 kg) compared with controls (Table 12). We found low SOE that switching to or adding adjunctive aripiprazole, adding the anticonvulsant medications topiramate and zonisamide, or adding metformin yield small to moderate weight loss. Nizatidine, an antihistamine, did not show any consistent effect on weight (low SOE). The SOE was insufficient for all other interventions. To put these weight loss changes in context, clinically important change in weight of 5 to 10 percent of body mass significantly reduces diabetes risk factors and cardiovascular disease risk in patients who have higher risk.[123,124] The strategies summarized in this report that found statically significant weight loss (i.e., behavioral interventions, adjunctive aripiprazole, anticonvulsants topiramate and zonisamide) yielded mean differences of 2 to 6 percent reductions in body weight over mean baseline weights.

The findings we report here for behavioral interventions and metformin are consistent with a recent review that examined treatments for obesity relevant to primary care.[125] Behaviorally based interventions resulted in a mean 3-kg greater weight loss than control over 12 to 18 months, with more treatment sessions associated with greater weight loss. In our review, no studies evaluated orlistat, an FDA-approved medication for the treatment of obesity that is also available without prescription at a lower dose. Orlistat is associated with approximately a 3-kilogram weight reduction over 12 to 18 months, but it must be used in conjunction with a low-fat diet.

Table 12. Summary SOE for KQ 1: Interventions for weight control

Outcome	Number of Studies (Subjects)	SOE Domains: ROB Consistency	SOE Domains: Directness Precision	SOE; Effect Estimate
Psychotropic Medications: Atomoxetine, Fluoxetine, Ramelteon, Adjunctive Aripiprazole				
Weight	4 (268)	Moderate NA[a]	Direct Imprecise	Insufficient; single studies showing no effect for atomoxetine, fluoxetine, ramelteon; small effects for amantadine and adjunctive aripiprazole
Physical function/ HRQOL	1 (207)	Low NA	Direct Imprecise	Insufficient; 1 study showing no positive effect
Adverse effects	1 (207)	Low NA	Direct Imprecise	Insufficient; 1 study reporting discontinuation due to adverse effects
Anticonvulsant Medications: Topiramate, Zonisamide				
Weight	3 (158)	Moderate Consistent	Direct Imprecise	Low; mean difference -5.1 kg (95% CI, -9.8 to -0.7)
Physical function/ HRQOL	1 (67)	Moderate NA	Direct Imprecise	Insufficient; positive effects on multiple scales for topiramate in a single study
Adverse effects	1 (42)	Low NA	Indirect Imprecise	Insufficient; only reported discontinuation due to adverse effects
Metformin				
Weight	5 (531)	Moderate Inconsistent	Direct Imprecise	Low; mean difference -4.1 kg (95% CI, -6.6 to -1.7)
Physical function/ HRQOL	No studies	NA	NA	Insufficient
Adverse effects	4 (475)	Low Consistent	Indirect Imprecise	Insufficient; inconsistent reporting of psychiatric adverse effects
Antihistamine: Nizatidine				
Weight	4 (286)	Moderate Inconsistent	Direct Precise	Low; mean difference -0.5 (95% CI, -1.3 to 0.3)
Physical function/ HRQOL	No studies	NA	NA	Insufficient
Adverse effects	1 (54)	Low NA	Indirect Imprecise	Insufficient; inconsistent reporting of major adverse effect of interest

Table 12. Summary SOE for KQ 1: Interventions for weight control (continued)

Outcome	Number of Studies (Subjects)	SOE Domains: ROB Consistency	SOE Domains: Directness Precision	SOE; Effect Estimate
Antipsychotic Switching				
Weight-aripiprazole	1 (133)	Moderate NA	Direct Imprecise	Low; mean difference -3.1 kg
Weight-olanzapine, quetiapine	3 (1203)	Moderate Consistent	Direct Imprecise	Insufficient for quetiapine, orally disintegrating and injectable olanzapine; single studies
Physical function/ HRQOL-aripiprizole	1 (133)	Moderate Inconsistent	Direct Imprecise	Insufficient
Physical function/ HrQOL-olanzapine, quetipaine	1 (149)	Low NA	Direct Imprecise	Insufficient; 1 study finding no difference with orally disintegrating olanzapine; no data for other drugs
Adverse effects-aripiprazole	1 (133)	Moderate NA	Indirect Imprecise	Insufficient
Adverse effects-olanzapine, quetiapine	3 (1203)	Moderate Consistent	Direct Imprecise	Insufficient; single studies for each drug
Behavioral Interventions				
Weight	11 (792)	Moderate Consistent	Direct Precise	Moderate Mean difference -3.1kg (-4.2 to -2.1)
Physical function/ HRQOL	1 (48)	High NA	Direct Imprecise	Insufficient
Adverse effects	2 (199)	Moderate Consistent	Direct Imprecise	Insufficient
Peer or Family Support Interventions				
All outcomes	No studies	NA	NA	Insufficient

CI = confidence interval; CVD = cardiovascular disease; HRQOL = health-related quality of life; kg = kilogram; NA = not applicable; OR = odds ratio; RCT = randomized controlled trial; ROB = risk of bias; SOE = strength of evidence
[a]Consistency rating does not apply where different drugs in the same general drug class are being summarized.

Key Question 2: Diabetes Control

We identified only seven trials that assessed the impact of behavioral and pharmacological interventions to address glucose control as measured by HbA1c in patients with SMI and elevated risk for CVD. Of these, only one study assessed patients with diabetes and glucose control directly;[105] the other six studies assessed HbA1c as a secondary outcome. Overall, we found insufficient evidence for all interventions (Table 13). Among populations without SMI who have diabetes, disease management programs[126] and metformin have been effective, as have lifestyle interventions for improving glucose control in people with diabetes or at risk of developing diabetes. Further, metformin is associated with decreased cardiovascular events compared with no treatment.[127] To place these findings in context, prospective trials have documented reduced rates of microvascular complications in patients with type 2 diabetes who are treated to lower glycemic targets.[128] In patients with newly diagnosed diabetes, these benefits were achieved with an average reduction in A1c of 0.9 percent.[129] A meta-analysis of trials in patients with established diabetes suggested that every 1 percent reduction in A1c may be associated with a 15-percent relative risk reduction in nonfatal myocardial infarction.[130] On average, oral hypoglycemic medications (e.g., metformin) are associated with approximately a one-percent decrease in HbA1c. These interventions may also translate to populations with SMI and warrant exploration.

Table 13. Summary SOE for KQ 2: Interventions for diabetes control (glucose)

Outcome	Number of Studies (Subjects)	SOE Domains: ROB Consistency	SOE Domains: Directness Precision	SOE; Effect Estimate
Psychotropic Medication: Ramelteon				
A1c	1 (20)	Moderate NA	Direct Imprecise	Insufficient; 1 small study showing small reduction in A1c
Physical function/ HRQOL	No studies	NA	NA	Insufficient
Adverse effects	1 (20)	Moderate NA	Indirect Imprecise	Insufficient
Anticonvulsant Medications				
All outcomes	No studies	NA	NA	Insufficient
Metformin				
A1c	2 (260)	High Inconsistent	Direct Imprecise	Insufficient; 2 studies, 1 using metformin with other medications in a treatment algorithm showing small reductions in A1c
Physical function/ HRQOL	No studies	NA	NA	Insufficient
Adverse effects	2 (260)	High Consistent	Direct Imprecise	Insufficient
Antipsychotic Switching: Olanzapine to Quetiapine, Aripiprazole, or Orally Disintegrating Olanzapine				
A1c	3 (497)	Low Consistent	Direct Precise	Moderate; range of mean difference 0 to -0.1
Physical function/ HRQOL	1 (215)	Low NA	Direct Imprecise	Insufficient; 1 study showing improvements in physical functioning
Adverse effects	3 (497)	Low Consistent	Direct Imprecise	Low; switching strategies had higher discontinuations, often due to psychiatric adverse effects
Behavioral Interventions				
A1c	2 (117)	Moderate Inconsistent	Direct Imprecise	Insufficient; range of mean difference -0.6 to 0
Physical function/ HRQOL	No studies	NA	NA	Insufficient
Adverse effects	1 (64)	Moderate NA	Direct Imprecise	Insufficient
Peer or Family Support Interventions				
All outcomes	No studies	NA	NA	Insufficient

CIb = confidence interval; CVD = cardiovascular disease; HRQOL = health-related quality of life; NA = not applicable; OR = odds ratio; RCT = randomized controlled trial; ROB = risk of bias; SOE = strength of evidence

Key Question 3: Lipid Control

No studies evaluated an intervention specifically designed to target lipid levels in patients with SMI who have dyslipidemia or are at risk for dyslipidemia. Behavioral interventions focusing on weight loss or diabetes management have no substantial effects on lipids. Small benefits were seen when aripiprazole was used as an adjunct or as an antipsychotic-switching strategy (low SOE), and single studies suggested possible benefit with ramelteon or topiramate. However, SOE was insufficient for all other interventions (Table 14). In contrast, low to moderate doses of statins are associated with a 20 to 40 percent reduction in LDL cholesterol.[131,132]

Table 14. Summary SOE for KQ 3: Interventions for lipid control

Outcome	Number of Studies (Subjects)	SOE Domains: ROB Consistency	SOE Domains: Directness Precision	SOE; Effect Estimate
Psychotropic Medications: Atomoxetine, Ramelteon, Adjunctive Aripiprazole				
Total cholesterol	2 (232)	Moderate NA[a]	Direct Imprecise	Insufficient; 1 study showing no effect on LDL cholesterol for atomoxetine, 1 study showing benefit on total cholesterol for ramelteon, 1 study showing benefit for adjunctive aripiprazole on total and LDL cholesterol
LDL cholesterol	3 (269)	Moderate NA[a]	Direct Imprecise	
Physical function/ HRQOL	1 (207)	Low NA	NA	Insufficient; 1 study showing no benefit
Adverse effects	2 (243)	Moderate NA[a]	Direct Imprecise	Insufficient; 1 study showed better mental health but more serious adverse events with adjunctive aripiprazole
Anticonvulsant Medications: Topiramate, Zonisamide				
Total cholesterol	1 (42)	Low NA	Direct Imprecise	Insufficient; 1 study showing moderate benefit (mean difference, 10.2 mg%) with topiramate on LDL; 1 study showing no effect with zonisamide
LDL cholesterol	2 (114)	Moderate Inconsistent	Direct Imprecise	
Physical function/ HRQOL	No studies	NA	NA	Insufficient
Adverse effects	No studies	NA	NA	Insufficient
Other Medications: Amantadine, Nizatidine				
Total cholesterol	2 (75)	Low to High NA[a]	Direct Imprecise	Insufficient; single studies for amantadine and nizatidine showing no effect
LDL cholesterol	2 (75)			
Physical function/ HRQOL	No studies	NA	NA	Insufficient
Adverse effects	1 (54)	Low NA	Indirect Imprecise	Insufficient
Antipsychotic Switching				
Total cholesterol	4 (1376)	Moderate Inconsistent	Direct Imprecise	Low for aripiprazole, insufficient for other antipsychotics; results varied by switching strategy. Only a switch to aripiprazole improved lipid values; switching to injectable olanzapine increased lipid values.
LDL cholesterol	4 (1376)			
Physical function/ HRQOL	1 (149)	Low NA	Direct Imprecise	Insufficient
Adverse effects	3 (1243)	Moderate Consistent	Indirect Imprecise	Low that moderate to large differences are not present for serious adverse events or discontinuations due to adverse events Insufficient for risk of psychiatric worsening

Table 14. Summary SOE for KQ 3: Interventions for lipid control (continued)

Outcome	Number of Studies (Subjects)	SOE Domains: ROB Consistency	SOE Domains: Directness Precision	SOE; Effect Estimate
Behavioral Interventions				
Total cholesterol	2 (99)	Moderate Consistent	Direct Imprecise	Insufficient
LDL cholesterol	3 (156)	Moderate Consistent	Indirect Imprecise	Insufficient; mean difference, 1.9 mg/dl (-6.1 to 9.9)
Physical function/ HRQOL	No studies	NA	NA	Insufficient
Adverse effects	1 (49)	High NA	Indirect Imprecise	Insufficient
Peer or family support interventions				
All outcomes	No studies	NA	NA	Insufficient

CI = confidence interval; CVD = cardiovascular disease; HRQOL = health-related quality of life; LDL = low-density lipoprotein; NA = not applicable; OR = odds ratio; RCT = randomized controlled trial; ROB = risk of bias; SOE = strength of evidence
[a]Consistency rating does not apply where different drugs in the same general drug class are being summarized.

Key Question 4: Multicondition Lifestyle Interventions

Few studies evaluated multicondition interventions, and these studies evaluated only a limited number of components (Table 15). Two studies evaluated multicomponent lifestyle interventions alone, and one evaluated switching from one of three second-generation antipsychotic medications to aripiprazole in combination with a structured diet and exercise program. None of these studies evaluated lifestyle interventions in combination with medications that directly address weight (e.g., orlistat), glucose (e.g., metformin), or lipids (e.g., statins). Studies reported each outcome separately without reporting an overall CVD risk such as the Framingham Risk Score. As described above, when adding or switching to aripiprazole, there is low SOE for a small benefit on weight, but the evidence is insufficient for overall CVD risk. The two multicomponent behavioral interventions did not have a positive effect on the individual CVD risk factors, although one of the two studies showed a large positive effect on health-related quality of life.

Table 15. Summary SOE for KQ 4: Multicondition lifestyle interventions

Outcome	Number of Studies (Subjects)	SOE Domains: ROB Consistency	SOE Domains: Directness Precision	SOE; Effect Estimate
Multicondition Interventions				
CVD risk	1 (41)	Moderate NA	Direct Imprecise	Insufficient; 1 study showing no positive effects
Physical function/ HRQOL	2 (245)	Low Inconsistent	Direct Imprecise	Insufficient; 2 studies showing no effect of multicomponent behavioral intervention but positive effects with switching to aripiprazole plus behavioral intervention
Adverse effects	1 (215)	Low NA	Direct Imprecise	Insufficient; greater discontinuation due to adverse effects and greater serious adverse effects in aripiprazole plus behavioral intervention

CVD = cardiovascular disease; HRQOL = health-related quality of life; NA = not applicable; ROB = risk of bias; SOE = strength of evidence

Findings in Relation to What Is Already Known

A number of high-quality systematic reviews have evaluated the comparative benefits and harms of antipsychotic medications.[133,134] However, these reviews focused on mental health outcomes and adverse effects, including adverse metabolic consequences, but not strategies for managing the adverse metabolic effects. Other reviews have identified effective treatments for CVD risk factors such as obesity, tobacco use, and hyperlipidemia in *general populations* or in *adults at increased risk for CVD*.[125,135,136] We specifically excluded from our review evaluations of general health advice, smoking cessation interventions, and models that provide integrated mental health–general medical care because these topics had been the subject of recent high-quality reviews in patients with SMI.[35-39] Tsoi et al.[35,36] found that bupropion more than doubled the rate of smoking abstinence in smokers with schizophrenia without jeopardizing their mental state. There were few studies of other smoking cessation treatments (including nicotine replacement therapy) and no evidence of benefit for these other treatments. In contrast, Tosh et al.[37] found a small number of RCTs evaluating general physical health advice for patients with SMI, and no clear benefit on health outcomes. Bradford et al.[39] found moderately strong evidence that integrated mental health–general medical care improves preventive services, including cardiovascular screening, but limited and inconsistent effects on physical functioning and CVD risk factors.

Our results complement prior reports by examining a broad array of interventions for patients at increased risk for worsening health outcomes due to CVD risk factors such as obesity, hyperlipidemia, diabetes mellitus, or chronic administration of antipsychotic medication that negatively impacts metabolic parameters. Earlier narrative and systematic reviews have focused primarily on behavioral interventions for weight control in patients with schizophrenia or who were on antipsychotic medications.[52,68,76,77,137-139] These reviews used differing eligibility criteria, with some including observational designs. Therefore, the number of studies included varied widely, ranging from 14 to 30. Despite the differences in methods, the conclusions of these reviews are largely consistent with our findings that behavioral interventions are associated with small improvements in weight. Some recent qualitative syntheses identified (1) interventions adapted to individuals with SMI, (2) durations of at least 3 months, and (3) incorporation of both education and activity-based approaches as associated with greater effects.[52,138] These findings are tempered by the small number of studies and indirect comparisons. Our review builds on these findings by identifying clear omissions in treatments that are known to be effective in non-SMI populations, including guideline-concordant care, and promising treatment strategies such as aripiprazole, metformin, and topiramate, which deserve further investigation.

Applicability

The positive effects of interventions do not always translate well to usual practice—where clinician training, clinical setting, system resources, and patient characteristics may vary importantly from trial conditions. In our review, only 15 of 35 trials were conducted in the United States, and most studies (n=21) were classified as efficacy studies and were relatively short in duration. Studies typically enrolled midlife adults; none specifically enrolled older adults. Women, as well as racial minorities, were well represented overall but underrepresented for some specific comparisons. Most studies were conducted in mental health outpatient settings, typical of the principal locus of medical care for patients with SMI; none were conducted in patient-centered medical homes or in settings that integrated mental health with general medical services. None were classified as effectiveness studies, but for many interventions, initial studies are justifiably designed to answer the question, Can it work under ideal conditions?—before moving to a test of effectiveness. Probably the most important constraint on applicability is the inconsistent reporting of the CVD-related outcomes of interest and the nearly total lack of reporting (only reported in one study) for overall CVD risk indices (e.g., Framingham Risk Score). Understanding intervention effects on overall CVD risk would, arguably, be reported as effects on CVD risk indices,[140] cardiovascular events (e.g., stroke, myocardial infarction) or CVD-related mortality—all of which were missing from the included trials except for one that reported CVD risk indices.[121]

Implications for Clinical and Policy Decisionmaking

The U.S. Preventive Services Task Force makes recommendations for CVD screening in adults, including blood pressure[141] and tobacco use,[142] screening for diabetes in patients with elevated blood pressure,[143] and lipid screening in midlife adults or young adults at increased risk for CVD.[144] Increasing guideline-concordant care for individuals with SMI—given the current lack of evidence for SMI-specific interventions—could be considered a starting point for minimizing CVD risk in patients with SMI. These guidelines for the general population should then be modified to consider the special risks for patients with SMI. In 2004, the American Diabetes Association and American Psychiatric Association issued consensus guidelines[145] for screening and monitoring of patients taking antipsychotic drugs. These guidelines recommended baseline monitoring to include a family history, BMI, waist circumference, blood pressure, fasting plasma glucose, and fasting lipid profile as well as followup monitoring of weight, fasting glucose, lipid levels, and blood pressure. Diabetes screening guidelines have since been updated to include the HbA1c as an appropriate measure to screen for diabetes mellitus.[146] Although screening and monitoring are addressed well by current guidelines, the American Psychiatric Association guidelines for schizophrenia provide only general advice for managing adverse effects of antipsychotic medication, such as helping the patient tolerate the adverse effect, treating the comorbid condition, or considering a change in the psychotropic medication to an alternative with less potential to induce side effects.

Our review, together with other reviews on interventions to decrease CVD risk in patients with or without SMI, suggests a few actionable strategies and others requiring further study. For weight control, moderate evidence supports behavioral interventions, and more limited evidence supports metformin, topiramate, or aripiprazole as an adjunctive or antipsychotic-switching strategy. All of these interventions yield small to moderate effects, and the benefits must be weighed against the potential harms. Because only limited data on harms were reported in the trials examined, data from non-SMI populations should be incorporated into decisionmaking. For example, metformin requires careful patient selection and monitoring of renal function due to the small risk of lactic acidosis.[147] Topiramate has an increased risk of paraesthesia, taste impairment, and psychomotor disturbances.[148] Data are much more limited for effects on average glucose control or lipid levels in patients at increased risk. The antihistamine nizatidine was not effective for any CVD risk factor and is unlikely to be a useful treatment. Other reviews identify bupropion as the best supported treatment for smoking cessation;[35,36] nicotine replacement therapy is effective in non-SMI populations but has not been adequately studied in patients with schizophrenia, bipolar disorder or psychotic depression. Other reviews identified tailored mood management in patients with depressive symptoms[149,150] and behavioral support interventions in individuals with mental illness as potentially effective.[151] Although the evidence is limited, the meta-finding is that, of the interventions tested in SMI populations to date, effects on intermediate outcomes (e.g., weight) are similar to the effects found in the general population.

Physicians take an oath of *primum non nocere*: First do no harm. The American Psychiatric Association's 2004 guidance follows this principle, recommending a response to adverse medication effects by considering a change in the psychotropic medication to an alternative with less potential to induce side effects. When treating emergent metabolic abnormalities that temporally follow medication treatment, this approach is rational, but existing data show only small improvements in the cardiovascular outcomes of interest. Other high-quality systematic reviews have addressed the comparative efficacy of antipsychotics and identified few differences in short-term efficacy between second-generation antipsychotics; clozapine reduced suicides and suicidal behavior, and clozapine and olanzapine had lower rates of discontinuation. Olanzapine resulted in greater weight gain and increased risk of new onset diabetes.[134] In patients who have responded well to psychotropic medication, a change in treatment carries the risk of symptom-worsening, an outcome not consistently reported in the studies reviewed. Further, antipsychotic-switching strategies have not been tested directly against treatments that target the metabolic abnormality directly (e.g., statin for hyperlipidemia) or multimodal strategies that include medication switching and lifestyle interventions. For some medications, interactions with psychotropic medications (e.g., thiazide diuretics and lithium) may limit effectiveness. Despite this caution, and in the absence of direct evidence in patients with SMI, treatments established as effective in non-SMI populations are a logical choice to treat risk factors for CVD in SMI populations until better evidence is available.

Studies of guideline adherence show significant gaps between current practice and recommendations for CVD risk screening and followup.[152] Studies show screening rates ranging from about 10 to 26 percent for lipids and 22 to 52 percent for glucose.[153-156] Data on monitoring of these risk factors in patients treated with second-generation antipsychotics are more limited but also show gaps between guidelines and practice. Assessment and monitoring is only a first step. When abnormalities are detected, they must be addressed, either by the mental health professional or by a general medicine clinician. Integrated mental health–general medical care has shown promise as the optimal way to deliver this care, and the current move to medical homes has the potential to make this type of care more readily available. Unfortunately, few medical home models to date have explicitly included mental health care.[157] Until integrated care is better established and more readily available, there are a number of implementation strategies to consider when a change to a metabolically more neutral antipsychotic is not sufficient to address elevated CVD risk factors. When patients have access to both mental health specialty care and general medical care, it is important that these clinicians coordinate care across issues that may impact both physical and mental health. For example, general medical providers may be aware of the adverse metabolic effects of some psychotropics but are appropriately hesitant to adjust these medications. Coordinating care with the mental health professional about roles and specific strategies for addressing CVD risk factors has the potential to improve care and clinical outcomes.

When general medical care is unavailable, one pragmatic strategy to consider is an expanded role for psychiatrists. Weight and blood pressure screening and monitoring are low-cost measures, requiring minimal time and office equipment. For patients without access to general medical care, psychiatrists could incorporate these activities into their usual clinical practice. Treating hyperlipidemia with statins is only slightly more difficult. The FDA and guidelines groups have recently revised recommendations; periodic transaminase monitoring is no longer recommended. In addition, some authors have made a strong case for fixed-dose statins that would further decrease the need for ongoing monitoring of lipid levels.[158] Thus, psychiatrists would need only to follow NCEP-III guidelines for when to initiate treatment (and readily available Web and smartphone-based applications facilitate quick access to these guidelines) and consider potential drug-drug interactions, which are relatively few.

Limitations of the Comparative Effectiveness Review Process

Our study has a number of strengths, including a protocol-driven review, a comprehensive search, careful quality assessment, and rigorous synthesis methods. Our report, and the literature, also has limitations. There were substantial limitations in the literature. First, the number of studies is small, many had design limitations affecting the validity of findings, and the range of interventions evaluated was limited. Further, descriptions of the interventions were often inadequate to permit replication. Second, there were few studies in certain populations of high interest (e.g., depression with psychosis, bipolar disorder). Third, the range of outcomes was limited, including infrequent reporting of overall CVD risk, physical functioning, and outcomes related to worsening of psychiatric status. Limitations in the number and reporting of studies precluded any analyses of variability in treatment effects by patient characteristics.

Our review methods also had limitations. Our study was limited to English-language publications. However, the likelihood of identifying relevant data unavailable from English-language sources is low. Although the definition of SMI includes major depression with persistent impairment in multiple areas of functioning, this concept is not specified with search terms, and thus we used the operational definition of psychotic depression. Also, only one study was specifically designed to address diabetes, and no studies directly targeted dyslipidemia. Thus, results for those CVD risks were culled from secondary outcome assessments of primarily weight management interventions. If a trial provided information on weight, glucose, and lipid control, these results were organized for the outcomes across KQ 1 through KQ 3 to reduce redundancy of reporting. However, we reported on adverse events and health-related quality of life for each study or class of intervention in each chapter. We excluded studies whose primary goal was to control psychiatric symptoms, thus, potentially excluding some antipsychotic trials that had relevant outcomes information, particularly related to adverse events. However, the recent DERP report[134] and AHRQ report[133] on the comparative effectiveness of antipsychotics provide a robust review of these outcomes as they pertain to adverse events of these treatments. Although we attempted to evaluate the impact of effectiveness versus efficacy studies, the small number of studies overall and lack of effectiveness studies made this analysis unfeasible.

Research Gaps

We used the framework recommended by Robinson et al.[159] to identify gaps in evidence and classify why these gaps exist. This approach considers PICOTS (population, intervention, comparator, outcomes, timing, and setting) to identify gaps and classifies gaps as due to (1) insufficient or imprecise information, (2) biased information; (3) inconsistency or unknown consistency, and (4) not the right information. In addition, we considered studies in progress identified from ClinicalTrials.gov when making recommendations for future research. Gaps and recommendations are presented in Table 16.

The list of gaps in evidence is long and one might reasonably ask which gaps have the highest priority. A full discussion of methods to establish a prioritized research agenda is beyond the scope of this report, but we suggest some general principles as applied to the population of adults with SMI. Most groups[160] advocate input from multiple stakeholders and consideration of issues such as the burden of disease (incorporating prevalence and impact on health), the availability of existing treatment options, the likelihood that the new intervention will substantially improve outcomes, practice variation and health disparities, and the feasibility of implementing effective interventions with existing resources. Specific research questions can be evaluated quantitatively, using value-of-information analysis, which employs Bayesian methods to estimate the potential benefits of gathering more information through research.[161] A recent AHRQ white paper used a multiple-stakeholder consensus process to identify patient-centered outcomes research priorities for serious mental illness.[162] This report identified 21 themes—ranging from retooling universities and education to specific treatment approaches. Conducting comparative effectiveness studies of interventions targeting modifiable risk factors such as tobacco abuse, physical exercise, and nutrition was identified as a research priority.

A second consideration in research prioritization is to identify research designs that are best suited to address the evidence gap. Randomized controlled trials are less susceptible to bias but are typically more expensive and slower to yield results than observational studies. Several studies[163,164] have compared interventions evaluated in both observational and randomized trials, showing high levels of concordance—but there have been notable exceptions. For example, vitamin E and conjugated estrogens appeared cardioprotective in observational studies, but RCTs did not show benefit.[165-167]

We suggest that observational designs may be particularly appropriate for these applications: (1) evaluating interventions proven effective in non-SMI populations, (2) testing the *effectiveness* of interventions demonstrated efficacious in tightly controlled trials, and (3) formulating hypotheses to be tested in RCTs. RCTs may be particularly useful for interventions specifically tailored for SMI populations and for drugs, or drug strategies (e.g., antipsychotic switching), that are used primarily in this population. Although we recommend multicenter RCTs to address some evidence gaps, we are aware that there are particular challenges to conducting RCTs in this population. For example, individuals with SMI have been routinely excluded from large cardiovascular trials—limiting opportunities to participate in research. Also, behavioral interventions may be affected by limited access to healthy foods or opportunities for exercise because many individuals with SMI are in lower socioeconomic status groups. Symptoms of mental illness and effects on cognition may make it difficult for individuals with SMI to fully participate in planned interventions. Some important outcomes, such as cardiovascular events, may take large sample sizes and long followup periods to evaluate.

Table 16. Evidence gaps and future research for adults with SMI

	Evidence Gap	Reason	Type of Studies to Consider
Patients	Limited data for patients with conditions other than schizophrenia	Insufficient information	Single and multisite RCTs Quasi-experimental or clinical records-based observational studies
Patients	No data in older adults who have more comorbid medical illness	Insufficient information	Single and multisite RCTs Quasi-experimental or clinical records-based observational studies
Patients	Few studies of ethnic and racial minorities	Insufficient information	Single and multisite RCTs Quasi-experimental or clinical records-based observational studies
Interventions	No interventions evaluating peer and family support interventions	Insufficient information	Single and multisite RCTs
Interventions	No studies on the effects of the most recently approved second-generation antipsychotics such as paliperidone, iloperidone, asenapine, and lurasidone	Insufficient information	Single and multisite RCTs Quasi-experimental or clinical records-based observational studies
Interventions	Limited evidence about the benefits and harms of switching from one antipsychotic to another on metabolic parameters	Insufficient information	Secondary analyses of existing studies such as the CATIE trial or large observational datasets
Interventions	No studies comparing optimized antipsychotic management (e.g., start with or switch to drugs with more favorable metabolic profiles) with continuing current antipsychotics in responders and treating adverse metabolic effects directly using treatments (e.g., statins) with known efficacy	Insufficient information	Single and multisite RCTs Quasi-experimental studies
Interventions	Few multimodal interventions (e.g., robust behavioral and pharmacological treatments) and few multicondition interventions (interventions that address multiple CVD risk factors)	Insufficient information	Single and multisite RCTs
Interventions	Few evaluations of smoking cessation interventions other than bupropion[a]	Insufficient information	Single and multisite RCTs Quasi-experimental or clinical records-based observational studies
Interventions	Few studies evaluating integrated mental health and general medical care[a]	Insufficient information	Single and multisite RCTs Quasi-experimental or clinical records-based observational studies
Interventions	Uncertainty about the key characteristics of successful behavioral interventions (e.g., tailoring, dose, duration, delivery mode, individual vs. group)	Insufficient information Not the right information	Improved intervention reporting Single and multisite RCTs Systematic reviews
Interventions	Uncertainty about the details of the intervention	Not the right information	Manuals provided to promote replication/implementation of successful interventions
Interventions	Interventions to improve guideline concordant care	Insufficient information	Single and multisite RCTs Quasi-experimental studies
Comparators	Few studies comparing two active interventions	Insufficient information	Single and multisite RCTs comparing effective treatments Quasi-experimental or clinical records-based observational studies

Table 16. Evidence gaps and future research for adults with SMI (continued)

	Evidence Gap	Reason	Type of Studies to Consider
Outcomes	Uncertain effects on overall CVD risk or cardiovascular events	Insufficient information	Risk indices (e.g., Framingham Risk Score) and/or cardiovascular events used as outcome measures
	Intervention adherence	Insufficient information	Improved study reporting
	Uncertainty about adverse effects on mental health status and other serious adverse effects, specifically in individuals with SMI	Insufficient information	Studies that define and report the proportion of patients for whom mental health status worsens Improved reporting of adverse effects
Timing	Few studies with outcomes measured beyond 6 months	Insufficient information	RCTs with longer term followup Quasi-experimental or observational studies
Setting	Lack of studies designed to evaluate "real world" effects of the intervention (effectiveness studies)	Insufficient information	RCTs or quasi-experimental studies with broad inclusion criteria, conducted in community practices, with long-term followup and which include clinically important outcomes such as physical functioning, cardiovascular events, and adverse events Improved reporting of efficacy–effectiveness characteristics

CATIE = Clinical Antipsychotic Trials in Intervention Effectiveness; CVD = cardiovascular disease; RCT = randomized controlled trial; SMI = serious mental illness

[a]Research gaps from prior high-quality systematic reviews that were identified during the topic refinement phase of this review and are described briefly in this report.

Conclusions

In summary, individuals with SMI are at risk for increased CVD—in part due to health behaviors, direct effects of the illness, and adverse effects from some treatments. Prior reviews identified bupropion as effective for smoking cessation, and integrated general medical and mental health care as effective for cardiovascular screening. In our review, surprisingly few studies addressed one or more CVD risk factors in patients with SMI, and most studies were skewed toward efficacy trials. Behavioral interventions, switching to or adding adjunctive aripiprazole, adding anticonvulsant medications topiramate and zonisamide, or adding metformin yield small to moderate weight loss compared with controls. We found insufficient evidence to support any strategy to control glucose. We found limited support of behavioral interventions focusing on weight loss or diabetes management or lipid control; SOE was insufficient for all other interventions. We found no studies testing a number of important interventions (e.g., orlistat, statins) known to be effective in non-SMI populations. Comparative effectiveness trials are needed that test multimodal strategies, known effective agents in non-SMI population (e.g., statins), and antipsychotic management strategies. However, in the absence of evidence for SMI-specific interventions, guideline-concordant care for individuals with SMI may help mitigate the unequal burden of CVD that SMI populations sustain.

References

1. National Institute of Mental Health. Statistics. www.nimh.nih.gov/statistics/index.shtml. Accessed June 22, 2012.

2. National Institute of Mental Health. Statistics. Schizophrenias. www.nimh.nih.gov/statistics/1SCHIZ.shtml. Accessed June 22, 2012.

3. Epstein J., Barker P, Vorburger M, et al. Serious mental illness and its co-occurrence with substance use disorders, 2002 (DHHS Publication No. SMA 04-3905, Analytic Series A-24). Rockville, MD: Substance Abuse and Mental Health Services Administration, Office of Applied Studies. www.samhsa.gov/data/CoD/CoD.pdf. Accessed June 22, 2012.

4. Chang C-K, Hayes R, Broadbent M, et al. All-cause mortality among people with serious mental illness (SMI), substance use disorders, and depressive disorders in southeast London: a cohort study. BMC Psychiatry. 2010;10(1):77. PMID: 20920287.

5. Brown AS, Birthwhistle J. Excess mortality of mental illness. Br J Psychiatry. 1996;169(3):383-4. PMID: 8879735.

6. Hsu JH, Chien IC, Lin CH, et al. Incidence of diabetes in patients with schizophrenia: a population-based study. Can J Psychiatry. 2011;56(1):19-26. PMID: 21324239.

7. Dixon L, Weiden P, Delahanty J, et al. Prevalence and correlates of diabetes in national schizophrenia samples. Schizophr Bull. 2000;26(4):903-12. PMID: 11087022.

8. van Winkel R, De Hert M, Van Eyck D, et al. Prevalence of diabetes and the metabolic syndrome in a sample of patients with bipolar disorder. Bipolar Disord. 2008;10(2):342-8. PMID: 18271914.

9. Bresee LC, Majumdar SR, Patten SB, et al. Prevalence of cardiovascular risk factors and disease in people with schizophrenia: a population-based study. Schizophr Res. 2010;117(1):75-82. PMID: 20080392.

10. Weiner M, Warren L, Fiedorowicz JG. Cardiovascular morbidity and mortality in bipolar disorder. Ann Clin Psychiatry. 2011;23(1):40-7. PMID: 21318195.

11. Kilbourne AM, Morden NE, Austin K, et al. Excess heart-disease-related mortality in a national study of patients with mental disorders: identifying modifiable risk factors. Gen Hosp Psychiatry. 2009;31(6):555-63. PMID: 19892214.

12. Miller BJ, Paschall CB, 3rd, Svendsen DP. Mortality and medical comorbidity among patients with serious mental illness. Psychiatr Serv. 2006;57(10):1482-7. PMID: 17035569.

13. Fagiolini A, Goracci A. The effects of undertreated chronic medical illnesses in patients with severe mental disorders. J Clin Psychiatry. 2009;70 Suppl 3:22-9. PMID: 19570498.

14. Ryan MC, Collins P, Thakore JH. Impaired fasting glucose tolerance in first-episode, drug-naive patients with schizophrenia. Am J Psychiatry. 2003;160(2):284-9. PMID: 12562574.

15. Kupfer DJ. The increasing medical burden in bipolar disorder. JAMA. 2005;293(20):2528-30. PMID: 15914754.

16. McCreadie RG. Diet, smoking and cardiovascular risk in people with schizophrenia: descriptive study. Br J Psychiatry. 2003;183:534-9. PMID: 14645025.

17. McElroy SL. Obesity in patients with severe mental illness: overview and management. J Clin Psychiatry. 2009;70 Suppl 3:12-21. PMID: 19570497.

18. Fountoulakis KN, Siamouli M, Panagiotidis P, et al. Obesity and smoking in patients with schizophrenia and normal controls: a case-control study. Psychiatry Res. 2010;176(1):13-6. PMID: 20079934.

19. Brown S, Birtwistle J, Roe L, et al. The unhealthy lifestyle of people with schizophrenia. Psychol Med. 1999;29(3):697-701. PMID: 10405091.

20. Kilbourne AM, Rofey DL, McCarthy JF, et al. Nutrition and exercise behavior among patients with bipolar disorder. Bipolar Disord. 2007;9(5):443-52. PMID: 17680914.

21. Newcomer JW. Metabolic considerations in the use of antipsychotic medications: a review of recent evidence. J Clin Psychiatry. 2007;68 Suppl 1:20-7. PMID: 17286524.

22. Kendler KS, Gallagher TJ, Abelson JM, et al. Lifetime prevalence, demographic risk factors, and diagnostic validity of nonaffective psychosis as assessed in a US community sample. The National Comorbidity Survey. Arch Gen Psychiatry. 1996;53(11):1022-31. PMID: 8911225.

23. Viron MJ, Stern TA. The impact of serious mental illness on health and healthcare. Psychosomatics. 2010;51(6):458-65. PMID: 21051676.

24. Desai MM, Rosenheck RA, Druss BG, et al. Receipt of nutrition and exercise counseling among medical outpatients with psychiatric and substance use disorders. J Gen Intern Med. 2002;17(7):556-60. PMID: 12133146.

25. Druss BG, Rosenheck RA, Desai MM, et al. Quality of preventive medical care for patients with mental disorders. Med Care. 2002;40(2):129-36. PMID: 11802085.

26. Green JL, Gazmararian JA, Rask KJ, et al. Quality of diabetes care for underserved patients with and without mental illness: site of care matters. Psychiatr Serv. 2010;61(12):1204-10. PMID: 21123404.

27. Frayne SM, Halanych JH, Miller DR, et al. Disparities in diabetes care: impact of mental illness. Arch Intern Med. 2005;165(22):2631-8. PMID: 16344421.

28. Mitchell AJ, Lord O. Do deficits in cardiac care influence high mortality rates in schizophrenia? A systematic review and pooled analysis. J Psychopharmacol. 2010;24(4 Suppl):69-80. PMID: 20923922.

29. McGuire J, Gelberg L, Blue-Howells J, et al. Access to primary care for homeless veterans with serious mental illness or substance abuse: a follow-up evaluation of co-located primary care and homeless social services. Administration and Policy in Mental Health. 2009;36(4):255-64. PMID: 19280333.

30. Druss BG, Rohrbaugh RM, Levinson CM, et al. Integrated medical care for patients with serious psychiatric illness: a randomized trial. Arch Gen Psychiatry. 2001;58(9):861-8. PMID: 11545670.

31. Warner CH, Morganstein J, Rachal J, et al. Perceptions and practices of graduates of combined family medicine-psychiatry residency programs: a nationwide survey. Acad Psychiatry. 2007;31(4):297-303. PMID: 17626192.

32. Bradford DW, Kim MM, Braxton LE, et al. Access to medical care among persons with psychotic and major affective disorders. Psychiatr Serv. 2008;59(8):847-52. PMID: 18678680.

33. Druss BG, Zhao L, von Esenwein SA, et al. The Health and Recovery Peer (HARP) Program: a peer-led intervention to improve medical self-management for persons with serious mental illness. Schizophr Res. 2010;118(1-3):264-70. PMID: 20185272.

34. Peck MC, Scheffler RM. An analysis of the definitions of mental illness used in state parity laws. Psychiatr Serv. 2002;53(9):1089-95. PMID: 12221306.

35. Tsoi DT, Porwal M, Webster AC. Interventions for smoking cessation and reduction in individuals with schizophrenia. Cochrane Database Syst Rev. 2010(6):CD007253. PMID: 20556777.

36. Tsoi DT, Porwal M, Webster AC. Efficacy and safety of bupropion for smoking cessation and reduction in schizophrenia: systematic review and meta-analysis. Br J Psychiatry. 2010;196(5):346-53. PMID: 20435957.

37. Tosh G, Clifton A, Bachner M. General physical health advice for people with serious mental illness. Cochrane Database Syst Rev. 2011;2:CD008567. PMID: 21328308.

38. Tosh G, Clifton A, Mala S, et al. Physical health care monitoring for people with serious mental illness. Cochrane Database Syst Rev. 2010(3):CD008298. PMID: 20238365.

39. Bradford DW, Slubicki MN, McDuffie JR, et al. Effects of care models to improve general medical outcomes for individuals with serious mental illness. VA-ESP Project #09-010; [In press.].

40. Agency for Healthcare Research and Quality. Methods Guide for Effectiveness and Comparative Effectiveness Reviews. Rockville, MD: Agency for Healthcare Research and Quality. www.effectivehealthcare.ahrq.gov/index.cfm/search-for-guides-reviews-and-reports/?pageaction=displayproduct&productid=318. Accessed June 12, 2012.

41. Moher D, Liberati A, Tetzlaff J, et al. Preferred Reporting Items for Systematic Reviews and Meta-Analyses: The PRISMA Statement. PLoS Med. 2009;6(7):e1000097. PMID: 19621072.

42. Anonymous. Evidence-based Practice Center Systematic Review Protocol. Project Title: Strategies To Improve Cardiovascular Risk Factors in People With Serious Mental Illness: A Comparative Effectiveness Review. www.effectivehealthcare.ahrq.gov/index.cfm/search-for-guides-reviews-and-reports/?productid=933&pageaction=displayproduct. Accessed June 22, 2012.

43. Agius M, Davis A, Gilhooley M, et al. What do large scale studies of medication in schizophrenia add to our management strategies? Psychiatr Danub. 2010;22(2):323-8. PMID: 20562774.

44. Allison DB, Mentore JL, Heo M, et al. Antipsychotic-induced weight gain: a comprehensive research synthesis. Am J Psychiatry. 1999;156(11):1686-96. PMID: 10553730.

45. Alvarez-Jimenez M, Hetrick SE, Gonzalez-Blanch C, et al. Non-pharmacological management of antipsychotic-induced weight gain: systematic review and meta-analysis of randomised controlled trials. Br J Psychiatry. 2008;193(2):101-7. PMID: 18669990.

46. Banham L, Gilbody S. Smoking cessation in severe mental illness: what works? Addiction. 2010;105(7):1176-89. PMID: 20491721.

47. Barkhof E, Meijer CJ, de Sonneville LM, et al. Interventions to improve adherence to antipsychotic medication in patients with schizophrenia-A review of the past decade. Eur Psychiatry. 2011. PMID: 21561742.

48. Beynon S, Soares-Weiser K, Woolacott N, et al. Pharmacological interventions for the prevention of relapse in bipolar disorder: a systematic review of controlled trials. J Psychopharmacol. 2009;23(5):574-91. PMID: 18635701.

49. Bradshaw T, Lovell K, Harris N. Healthy living interventions and schizophrenia: a systematic review. J Adv Nurs. 2005;49(6):634-54. PMID: 15737224.

50. Bushe CJ, Bradley AJ, Doshi S, et al. Changes in weight and metabolic parameters during treatment with antipsychotics and metformin: do the data inform as to potential guideline development? A systematic review of clinical studies. Int J Clin Pract. 2009;63(12):1743-61. PMID: 19840151.

51. Bushe CJ, Leonard BE. Blood glucose and schizophrenia: a systematic review of prospective randomized clinical trials. J Clin Psychiatry. 2007;68(11):1682-90. PMID: 18052561.

52. Cabassa LJ, Ezell JM, Lewis-Fernandez R. Lifestyle interventions for adults with serious mental illness: a systematic literature review. Psychiatr Serv. 2010;61(8):774-82. PMID: 20675835.

53. Citrome L, Holt RI, Walker DJ, et al. Weight gain and changes in metabolic variables following olanzapine treatment in schizophrenia and bipolar disorder. Clin Drug Investig. 2011;31(7):455-82. PMID: 21495734.

54. Citrome L. A review of aripiprazole in the treatment of patients with schizophrenia or bipolar I disorder. Neuropsychiatr Dis Treat. 2006;2(4):427-43. PMID: 19412492.

55. Ellinger LK, Ipema HJ, Stachnik JM. Efficacy of metformin and topiramate in prevention and treatment of second-generation antipsychotic-induced weight gain. Ann Pharmacother. 2010;44(4):668-79. PMID: 20233913.

56. Faulkner G, Cohn T, Remington G. Interventions to reduce weight gain in schizophrenia. Cochrane Database Syst Rev. 2007(1):CD005148. PMID: 17253540.

57. Karagianis J, Hoffmann VP, Arranz B, et al. Orally disintegrating olanzapine and potential differences in treatment-emergent weight gain. Hum Psychopharmacol. 2008;23(4):275-81. PMID: 18338426.

58. Komossa K, Rummel-Kluge C, Schmid F, et al. Quetiapine versus other atypical antipsychotics for schizophrenia. Cochrane Database Syst Rev. 2010(1):CD006625. PMID: 20091600.

59. Komossa K, Rummel-Kluge C, Hunger H, et al. Sertindole versus other atypical antipsychotics for schizophrenia. Cochrane Database Syst Rev. 2009(2):CD006752. PMID: 19370652.

60. Kreyenbuhl J, Buchanan RW, Dickerson FB, et al. The Schizophrenia Patient Outcomes Research Team (PORT): updated treatment recommendations 2009. Schizophr Bull. 2010;36(1):94-103. PMID: 19955388.

61. Leucht S, Kissling W, Davis JM. Second-generation antipsychotics for schizophrenia: can we resolve the conflict? Psychol Med. 2009;39(10):1591-602. PMID: 19335931.

62. Lipkovich I, Jacobson JG, Caldwell C, et al. Early predictors of weight gain risk during treatment with olanzapine: analysis of pooled data from 58 clinical trials. Psychopharmacol Bull. 2009;42(4):23-39. PMID: 20581791.

63. Mukundan A, Faulkner G, Cohn T, et al. Antipsychotic switching for people with schizophrenia who have neuroleptic-induced weight or metabolic problems. Cochrane Database Syst Rev. 2010(12):CD006629. PMID: 21154372.

64. Praharaj SK, Jana AK, Goyal N, et al. Metformin for olanzapine-induced weight gain: a systematic review and meta-analysis. Br J Clin Pharmacol. 2011;71(3):377-82. PMID: 21284696.

65. Rege S. Antipsychotic induced weight gain in schizophrenia:mechanisms and management. Aust N Z J Psychiatry. 2008;42(5):369-81. PMID: 18473255.

66. Rummel-Kluge C, Komossa K, Schwarz S, et al. Head-to-head comparisons of metabolic side effects of second generation antipsychotics in the treatment of schizophrenia: a systematic review and meta-analysis. Schizophr Res. 2010;123(2-3):225-33. PMID: 20692814.

67. Lee YJ, Jeong JH. A systematic review of metformin to limit weight-gain with atypical antipsychotics. J Clin Pharm Ther. 2011;36(5):537-545.

68. Verhaeghe N, De Maeseneer J, Maes L, et al. Effectiveness and cost-effectiveness of lifestyle interventions on physical activity and eating habits in persons with severe mental disorders: A systematic review. Int J Behav Nutr Phys Act. 2011;8.

69. Bjorkhem-Bergman L, Asplund AB, Lindh JD. Metformin for weight reduction in non-diabetic patients on antipsychotic drugs: A systematic review and meta-analysis. J Psychopharmacol. 2011;25(3):299-305.

70. Alvarez-Jimenez M. Tackling the physical consequences of psychosis and its treatment. Early Interv Psychiatry. 2010;4:17.

71. Strassnig M, Ganguli R. Weight loss interventions for patients with schizophrenia. Clin Schizophr Relat Psychoses. 2007;1(1):43-53.

72. Chue P, Stip E, Remington G, et al. Switching atypical antipsychotics: A review. Acta Neuropsychiatrica. 2004;16(6):301-313.

73. Bushe C, Leonard B. Association between atypical antipsychotic agents and type 2 diabetes: Review of prospective clinical data. Br J Psychiatry. 2004;184(SUPPL. 47):s87-s93.

74. Compton MT, Daumit GL, Druss BG. Cigarette smoking and overweight/obesity among individuals with serious mental illnesses: a preventive perspective. Harv Rev Psychiatry. 2006;14(4):212-22. PMID: 16912007.

75. Faulkner G, Soundy AA, Lloyd K. Schizophrenia and weight management: a systematic review of interventions to control weight. Acta Psychiatr Scand. 2003;108(5):324-32. PMID: 14551752.

76. Loh C, Meyer JM, Leckband SG. A comprehensive review of behavioral interventions for weight management in schizophrenia. Ann Clin Psychiatry. 2006;18(1):23-31. PMID: 16517450.

77. Gabriele JM, Dubbert PM, Reeves RR. Efficacy of behavioural interventions in managing atypical antipsychotic weight gain. Obes Rev. 2009;10(4):442-55. PMID: 19389059.

78. Newcomer JW, Haupt DW. The metabolic effects of antipsychotic medications. Can J Psychiatry. 2006;51(8):480-91. PMID: 16933585.

79. Faulkner G, Cohn T, Remington G. Interventions to reduce weight gain in schizophrenia. Schizophr Bull. 2007;33(3):654-6. PMID: 17449900.

80. Khan AY, Macaluso M, McHale RJ, et al. The adjunctive use of metformin to treat or prevent atypical antipsychotic-induced weight gain: a review. J Psychiatr Pract. 2010;16(5):289-96. PMID: 20859106.

81. Zimmermann U, Kraus T, Himmerich H, et al. Epidemiology, implications and mechanisms underlying drug-induced weight gain in psychiatric patients. J Psychiatr Res. 2003;37(3):193-220. PMID: 12650740.

82. Ganguli R. Behavioral therapy for weight loss in patients with schizophrenia. J Clin Psychiatry. 2007;68 Suppl 4:19-25. PMID: 17539696.

83. Gartlehner G, Hansen RA, Nissman D, et al. A simple and valid tool distinguished efficacy from effectiveness studies. J Clin Epidemiol. 2006;59(10):1040-8. PMID: 16980143.

84. Higgins JP, Thompson SG. Quantifying heterogeneity in a meta-analysis. Statistics in Medicine. 2002;21(11):1539-58. PMID: 12111919.

85. Begg CB, Mazumdar M. Operating characteristics of a rank correlation test for publication bias. Biometrics. 1994;50(4):1088-101. PMID: 7786990.

86. Owens DK, Lohr KN, Atkins D, et al. AHRQ series paper 5: Grading the strength of a body of evidence when comparing medical interventions—Agency for Healthcare Research and Quality and the Effective Health-Care Program. J Clin Epidemiol. 2010;63(5):513-23. PMID: 19595577.

87. Atkins D, Chang SM, Gartlehner G, et al. Assessing applicability when comparing medical interventions: AHRQ and the Effective Health Care Program. J Clin Epidemiol. 2011;64(11):1198-207. PMID: 21463926.

88. Alvarez-Jimenez M, Gonzalez-Blanch C, Vazquez-Barquero JL, et al. Attenuation of antipsychotic-induced weight gain with early behavioral intervention in drug-naive first-episode psychosis patients: A randomized controlled trial. J Clin Psychiatry. 2006;67(8):1253-60. PMID: 16965204.

89. Assuncao SS, Ruschel SI, Rosa Lde C, et al. Weight gain management in patients with schizophrenia during treatment with olanzapine in association with nizatidine. Rev Bras Psiquiatr. 2006;28(4):270-6. PMID: 17242805.

90. Atmaca M, Kuloglu M, Tezcan E, et al. Nizatidine for the treatment of patients with quetiapine-induced weight gain. Hum Psychopharmacol. 2004;19(1):37-40. PMID: 14716710.

91. Ball MP, Warren KR, Feldman S, et al. Placebo-controlled trial of atomoxetine for weight reduction in people with schizophrenia treated with clozapine or olanzapine. Clin Schizophr Relat Psychoses. 2011;5(1):17-25. PMID: 21459735.

92. Borba CP, Fan X, Copeland PM, et al. Placebo-controlled pilot study of ramelteon for adiposity and lipids in patients with schizophrenia. J Clin Psychopharmacol. 2011;31(5):653-8. PMID: 21869685.

93. Brar JS, Ganguli R, Pandina G, et al. Effects of behavioral therapy on weight loss in overweight and obese patients with schizophrenia or schizoaffective disorder. J Clin Psychiatry. 2005;66(2):205-12. PMID: 15705006.

94. Brown C, Goetz J, Hamera E. Weight loss intervention for people with serious mental illness: a randomized controlled trial of the RENEW program. Psychiatr Serv. 2011;62(7):800-2. PMID: 21724796.

95. Deberdt W, Lipkovich I, Heinloth AN, et al. Double-blind, randomized trial comparing efficacy and safety of continuing olanzapine versus switching to quetiapine in overweight or obese patients with schizophrenia or schizoaffective disorder. Ther Clin Risk Manag. 2008;4(4):713-20. PMID: 19209252.

96. Elmslie JL, Porter RJ, Joyce PR, et al. Carnitine does not improve weight loss outcomes in valproate-treated bipolar patients consuming an energy-restricted, low-fat diet. Bipolar Disord. 2006;8(5 Pt 1):503-7. PMID: 17042889.

97. Evans S, Newton R, Higgins S. Nutritional intervention to prevent weight gain in patients commenced on olanzapine: a randomized controlled trial. Aust N Z J Psychiatry. 2005;39(6):479-86. PMID: 15943650.

98. Fleischhacker WW, Heikkinen ME, Olie JP, et al. Effects of adjunctive treatment with aripiprazole on body weight and clinical efficacy in schizophrenia patients treated with clozapine: a randomized, double-blind, placebo-controlled trial. Int J Neuropsychopharmacol. 2010;13(8):1115-25. PMID: 20459883.

99. Gillhoff K, Gaab J, Emini L, et al. Effects of a multimodal lifestyle intervention on body mass index in patients with bipolar disorder: a randomized controlled trial. Prim Care Companion J Clin Psychiatry. 2010;12(5). PMID: 21274359.

100. Graham KA, Gu H, Lieberman JA, et al. Double-blind, placebo-controlled investigation of amantadine for weight loss in subjects who gained weight with olanzapine. Am J Psychiatry. 2005;162(9):1744-6. PMID: 16135638.

101. Hoffmann VP, Case M, Jacobson JG. Assessment of treatment algorithms including amantadine, metformin, and zonisamide for the prevention of weight gain with olanzapine: a randomized controlled open-label study. J Clin Psychiatry. 2012;73(2):216-23. PMID: 21672497.

102. Karagianis J, Grossman L, Landry J, et al. A randomized controlled trial of the effect of sublingual orally disintegrating olanzapine versus oral olanzapine on body mass index: the PLATYPUS Study. Schizophr Res. 2009;113(1):41-8. PMID: 19535229.

103. Kwon JS, Choi JS, Bahk WM, et al. Weight management program for treatment-emergent weight gain in olanzapine-treated patients with schizophrenia or schizoaffective disorder: A 12-week randomized controlled clinical trial. J Clin Psychiatry. 2006;67(4):547-53. PMID: 16669719.

104. Littrell KH, Hilligoss NM, Kirshner CD, et al. The effects of an educational intervention on antipsychotic-induced weight gain. J Nurs Scholarsh. 2003;35(3):237-41. PMID: 14562491.

105. McKibbin CL, Patterson TL, Norman G, et al. A lifestyle intervention for older schizophrenia patients with diabetes mellitus: a randomized controlled trial. Schizophr Res. 2006;86(1-3):36-44. PMID: 16842977.

106. Newcomer JW, Campos JA, Marcus RN, et al. A multicenter, randomized, double-blind study of the effects of aripiprazole in overweight subjects with schizophrenia or schizoaffective disorder switched from olanzapine. J Clin Psychiatry. 2008;69(7):1046-56. PMID: 18605811.

107. Wu RR, Zhao JP, Jin H, et al. Lifestyle intervention and metformin for treatment of antipsychotic-induced weight gain: a randomized controlled trial. JAMA. 2008;299(2):185-93. PMID: 18182600.

108. McDonnell DP, Kryzhanovskaya LA, Zhao F, et al. Comparison of metabolic changes in patients with schizophrenia during randomized treatment with intramuscular olanzapine long-acting injection versus oral olanzapine. Hum Psychopharmacol. 2011;26(6):422-433. PMID: 21823172.

109. Bustillo JR, Lauriello J, Parker K, et al. Treatment of weight gain with fluoxetine in olanzapine-treated schizophrenic outpatients. Neuropsychopharmacology. 2003;28(3):527-9. PMID: 12629532.

110. Atmaca M, Kuloglu M, Tezcan E, et al. Nizatidine treatment and its relationship with leptin levels in patients with olanzapine-induced weight gain. Hum Psychopharmacol. 2003;18(6):457-61. PMID: 12923824.

111. Cavazzoni P, Tanaka Y, Roychowdhury SM, et al. Nizatidine for prevention of weight gain with olanzapine: a double-blind placebo-controlled trial. Eur Neuropsychopharmacol. 2003;13(2):81-5. PMID: 12650950.

112. Nickel MK, Nickel C, Muehlbacher M, et al. Influence of topiramate on olanzapine-related adiposity in women: a random, double-blind, placebo-controlled study. J Clin Psychopharmacol. 2005;25(3):211-7. PMID: 15876898.

113. Khazaal Y, Fresard E, Rabia S, et al. Cognitive behavioural therapy for weight gain associated with antipsychotic drugs. Schizophr Res. 2007;91(1-3):169-77. PMID: 17306507.

114. Mauri M, Simoncini M, Castrogiovanni S, et al. A psychoeducational program for weight loss in patients who have experienced weight gain during antipsychotic treatment with olanzapine. Pharmacopsychiatry. 2008;41(1):17-23. PMID: 18203047.

115. McElroy SL, Winstanley E, Mori N, et al. A randomized, placebo-controlled study of zonisamide to prevent olanzapine-associated weight gain. J Clin Psychopharmacol. 2012;32(2):165-72. PMID: 22367654.

116. Carrizo E, Fernandez V, Connell L, et al. Extended release metformin for metabolic control assistance during prolonged clozapine administration: a 14 week, double-blind, parallel group, placebo-controlled study. Schizophr Res. 2009;113(1):19-26. PMID: 19515536.

117. Wang M, Tong JH, Zhu G, et al. Metformin for treatment of antipsychotic-induced weight gain: a randomized, placebo-controlled study. Schizophr Res. 2012;138(1):54-7. PMID: 22398127.

118. Wu RR, Jin H, Gao K, et al. Metformin for Treatment of Antipsychotic-Induced Amenorrhea and Weight Gain in Women With First-Episode Schizophrenia: A Double-Blind, Randomized, Placebo-Controlled Study. Am J Psychiatry. 2012;169(8):813-21. PMID: 22711171.

119. Narula PK, Rehan HS, Unni KE, et al. Topiramate for prevention of olanzapine associated weight gain and metabolic dysfunction in schizophrenia: a double-blind, placebo-controlled trial. Schizophr Res. 2010;118(1-3):218-23. PMID: 20207521.

120. Stroup TS, McEvoy JP, Ring KD, et al. A randomized trial examining the effectiveness of switching from olanzapine, quetiapine, or risperidone to aripiprazole to reduce metabolic risk: comparison of antipsychotics for metabolic problems (CAMP). Am J Psychiatry. 2011;168(9):947-56. PMID: 21768610.

121. Forsberg KA, Bjorkman T, Sandman PO, et al. Physical health--a cluster randomized controlled lifestyle intervention among persons with a psychiatric disability and their staff. Nord J Psychiatry. 2008;62(6):486-95. PMID: 18843564.

122. Skrinar GS, Huxley NA, Hutchinson DS, et al. The role of a fitness intervention on people with serious psychiatric disabilities. Psychiatr Rehabil J. 2005;29(2):122-7. PMID: 16268007.

123. Douketis JD, Macie C, Thabane L, et al. Systematic review of long-term weight loss studies in obese adults: clinical significance and applicability to clinical practice. Int J Obes (Lond). 2005;29(10):1153-67. PMID: 15997250.

124. Knowler WC, Barrett-Connor E, Fowler SE, et al. Reduction in the incidence of type 2 diabetes with lifestyle intervention or metformin. N Engl J Med. 2002;346(6):393-403. PMID: 11832527.

125. Leblanc ES, O'Connor E, Whitlock EP, et al. Effectiveness of primary care-relevant treatments for obesity in adults: a systematic evidence review for the U.S. Preventive Services Task Force. Ann Intern Med. 2011;155(7):434-47. PMID: 21969342.

126. Zaza S, Briss PA, Harris KW, et al. The guide to community preventive services: what works to promote health? New York: Oxford University; 2005.

127. Lamanna C, Monami M, Marchionni N, et al. Effect of metformin on cardiovascular events and mortality: a meta-analysis of randomized clinical trials. Diabetes Obes Metab. 2011;13(3):221-8. PMID: 21205121.

128. Inzucchi SE, Bergenstal RM, Buse JB, et al. Management of hyperglycemia in type 2 diabetes: a patient-centered approach: position statement of the American Diabetes Association (ADA) and the European Association for the Study of Diabetes (EASD). Diabetes Care. 2012;35(6):1364-79. PMID: 22517736.

129. UK Prospective Diabetes Study (UKPDS) Group. Intensive blood-glucose control with sulphonylureas or insulin compared with conventional treatment and risk of complications in patients with type 2 diabetes (UKPDS 33). Lancet. 1998;352(9131):837-53. PMID: 9742976.

130. Turnbull FM, Abraira C, Anderson RJ, et al. Intensive glucose control and macrovascular outcomes in type 2 diabetes. Diabetologia. 2009;52(11):2288-98. PMID: 19655124.

131. The Medical Letter. Drugs for Lipids. Treatment Guidelines from The Medical Letter. Issue 66. February 2008.

132. Thavendiranathan P, Bagai A, Brookhart MA, et al. Primary prevention of cardiovascular diseases with statin therapy: a meta-analysis of randomized controlled trials. Arch Intern Med. 2006;166(21):2307-13. PMID: 17130382.

133. Anonymous. Evidence-based Practice Center Systematic Review Protocol. Project Title: Comparative Effectiveness of First and Second Generation Antipsychotics in the Adult Population. effectivehealthcare.ahrq.gov/index.cfm/search-for-guides-reviews-and-reports/?pageaction=displayproduct&productid=583. Accessed June 22, 2012.

134. McDonagh M, Peterson K, Carson S, et al. Drug Effectiveness Review Project. Drug Class Review: Atypical Antipsychotic Drugs. Final Update 3. Oregon Evidence-based Practice Center. July 2010. derp.ohsu.edu/about/final-document-display.cfm. Accessed June 15, 2012. PMID: 21348048.

135. Cahill K, Stead LF, Lancaster T. Nicotine receptor partial agonists for smoking cessation. Cochrane Database of Systematic Reviews. 2011(2). PMID: ISI:000288616600005.

136. Anonymous. Evidence-based Practice Center Systematic Review Protocol. Project Title: Comparative Effectiveness of Approaches to Weight Maintenance in Adults. www.effectivehealthcare.ahrq.gov/index.cfm/search-for-guides-reviews-and-reports/?productid=824&pageaction=displayproduct. Accessed June 22, 2012.

137. Happell B, Davies C, Scott D. Health behaviour interventions to improve physical health in individuals diagnosed with a mental illness: a systematic review. Int J Ment Health Nurs. 2012;21(3):236-47. PMID: 22533331.

138. Bartels S, Desilets R. Health Promotion Programs for People with Serious Mental Illness (Prepared by the Dartmouth Health Promotion Research Team). Washington, D.C. SAMHSA-HRSA Center for Integrated Health Solutions. January 2012. www.integration.samhsa.gov/Health_Promotion_White_Paper_Bartels_Final_Document.pdf. Accessed September 17, 2012.

139. Wildes JE, Marcus MD, Fagiolini A. Obesity in patients with bipolar disorder: a biopsychosocial-behavioral model. J Clin Psychiatry. 2006;67(6):904-15. PMID: 16848650.

140. Edelman D, Oddone EZ, Liebowitz RS, et al. A multidimensional integrative medicine intervention to improve cardiovascular risk. J Gen Intern Med. 2006;21(7):728-34. PMID: 16808774.

141. U.S. Preventive Services Task Force. Screening for High Blood Pressure: U.S. Preventive Services Task Force Reaffirmation Recommendation Statement. AHRQ Publication No. 08-05105-EF-2, December 2007. First published in Ann Intern Med 2007:147-783-786. www.uspreventiveservicestaskforce.org/uspstf07/hbp/hbprs.htm. Accessed June 15, 2012.

142. U.S. Preventive Services Task Force. Counseling to Prevent Tobacco Use and Tobacco-Caused Disease Recommendation Statement. www.uspreventiveservicestaskforce.org/3rduspstf/tobacccoun/tobcounrs.htm. Accessed June 15, 2012.

143. Norris SL, Kansagara D, Bougatsos C, et al. Screening for Type 2 Diabetes: Update of 2003 Systematic Evidence Review for the U.S. Preventive Services Task Force. Evidence Synthesis No. 61. AHRQ Publication No. 08-05116-EF-1. Rockville, Maryland: Agency for Healthcare Research and Quality. June 2008. www.ncbi.nlm.nih.gov/books/NBK33981/. Accessed June 15, 2012.

144. Helfand M, Carson S. Screening for Lipid Disorders in Adults: Selective Update of 2001 U.S. Preventive Services Task Force Review. Evidence Synthesis No. 49. Rockville, MD: Agency for Healthcare Research and Quality, April 2008. AHRQ Publication no. 08-05114-EF-1. www.ncbi.nlm.nih.gov/books/NBK33494/. Accessed June 15, 2012.

145. American Diabetes Association. Consensus development conference on antipsychotic drugs and obesity and diabetes. Diabetes Care. 2004;27(2):596-601. PMID: ISI:000188739900043.

146. Standards of Medical Care in Diabetes-2012. Diabetes Care. 2012;35(1):S11-S63. PMID: ISI:000298772200002.

147. Salpeter S, Greyber E, Pasternak G, et al. Risk of fatal and nonfatal lactic acidosis with metformin use in type 2 diabetes mellitus. Cochrane Database Syst Rev. 2006(1):CD002967. PMID: 16437448.

148. Kramer CK, Leitao CB, Pinto LC, et al. Efficacy and safety of topiramate on weight loss: a meta-analysis of randomized controlled trials. Obes Rev. 2011;12(5):e338-47. PMID: 21438989.

149. Gierisch JM, Bastian LA, Calhoun PS, et al. Smoking cessation interventions for patients with depression: a systematic review and meta-analysis. J Gen Intern Med. 2012;27(3):351-60. PMID: 22038468.

150. Gierisch JM, Bastian LA, Calhoun PS, et al. Comparative Effectiveness of Smoking Cessation Treatments for Patients With Depression: A Systematic Review and Meta-analysis of the Evidence. VA-ESP Project #09-010; 2010.

151. Bryant J, Bonevski B, Paul C, et al. A systematic review and meta-analysis of the effectiveness of behavioural smoking cessation interventions in selected disadvantaged groups. Addiction. 2011;106(9):1568-85. PMID: 21489007.

152. Mitchell AJ, Delaffon V, Vancampfort D, et al. Guideline concordant monitoring of metabolic risk in people treated with antipsychotic medication: systematic review and meta-analysis of screening practices. Psychol Med. 2012;42(1):125-47. PMID: 21846426.

153. Haupt DW, Rosenblatt LC, Kim E, et al. Prevalence and predictors of lipid and glucose monitoring in commercially insured patients treated with second-generation antipsychotic agents. Am J Psychiatry. 2009;166(3):345-53. PMID: 19147694.

154. Morrato EH, Newcomer JW, Kamat S, et al. Metabolic screening after the American Diabetes Association's consensus statement on antipsychotic drugs and diabetes. Diabetes Care. 2009;32(6):1037-42. PMID: 19244091.

155. Morrato EH, Druss B, Hartung DM, et al. Metabolic testing rates in 3 state Medicaid programs after FDA warnings and ADA/APA recommendations for second-generation antipsychotic drugs. Arch Gen Psychiatry. 2010;67(1):17-24. PMID: 20048219.

156. Morrato EH, Druss BG, Hartung DM, et al. Small area variation and geographic and patient-specific determinants of metabolic testing in antipsychotic users. Pharmacoepidemiol Drug Saf. 2011;20(1):66-75. PMID: 21182154.

157. Williams JW, Jackson GL, Powers BJ, et al. Closing the Quality Gap Series: Revisiting the State of the Science. The Patient-Centered Medical Home. (Prepared by the Duke Evidence-based Practice Center under Contract No. 290-2007-10066-I.) Rockville, MD. Agency for Healthcare Research and Quality. [in press].

158. Hayward RA, Hofer TP, Vijan S. Narrative review: lack of evidence for recommended low-density lipoprotein treatment targets: a solvable problem. Ann Intern Med. 2006;145(7):520-30. PMID: 17015870.

159. Robinson KA, Saldanha IJ, Mckoy NA. Frameworks for Determining Research Gaps During Systematic Reviews. Methods Future Research Needs Report No. 2. (Prepared by the Johns Hopkins University Evidence-based Practice Center under Contract No. HHSA 290-2007-10061-I.) AHRQ Publication No. 11-EHC043-EF. Rockville, MD: Agency for Healthcare Research and Quality. June 2011. www.effectivehealthcare.ahrq.gov/reports/final.cfm. Accessed May 22, 2012.

160. Patient-Centered Outcomes Research Institute. Draft National Priorities for Research and Research Agenda. Version 1. January 23, 2012.

161. Myers E, McBroom AJ, Shen L, et al. Value-of-Information Analysis for Patient-Centered Outcomes Research Prioritization. Report prepared by the Duke Evidence-based Practice Center. Patient-Centered Outcomes Research Institute. March 2012.

162. Jonas D, Mansfield AJ, Curtis P, et al. Identifying Priorities for Patient-Centered Outcomes Research for Serious Mental Illness. Research White Paper. (Prepared by the RTI-UNC Institute Evidence-based Practice Center under Contract No. 290-2007-10056-I.) AHRQ Publication No. 11-EHC066-EF. Rockville, MD: Agency for Healthcare Research and Quality. September 2011. www.effectivehealthcare.ahrq.gov/reports/final.cfm.

163. Concato J, Shah N, Horwitz RI. Randomized, controlled trials, observational studies, and the hierarchy of research designs. N Engl J Med. 2000;342(25):1887-92. PMID: 10861325.

164. Ioannidis JP, Haidich AB, Pappa M, et al. Comparison of evidence of treatment effects in randomized and nonrandomized studies. JAMA. 2001;286(7):821-30. PMID: 11497536.

165. Sesso HD, Buring JE, Christen WG, et al. Vitamins E and C in the prevention of cardiovascular disease in men: the Physicians' Health Study II randomized controlled trial. JAMA. 2008;300(18):2123-33. PMID: 18997197.

166. Lee IM, Cook NR, Gaziano JM, et al. Vitamin E in the primary prevention of cardiovascular disease and cancer: the Women's Health Study: a randomized controlled trial. JAMA. 2005;294(1):56-65. PMID: 15998891.

167. Anderson GL, Limacher M, Assaf AR, et al. Effects of conjugated equine estrogen in postmenopausal women with hysterectomy: the Women's Health Initiative randomized controlled trial. JAMA. 2004;291(14):1701-12. PMID: 15082697.

Abbreviations

AHRQ	Agency for Healthcare Research and Quality
CI	confidence interval
CVD	cardiovascular disease
df	degree of freedom
HR	hazard ratio
HRQOL	health-related quality of life
kg	kilogram
KQ	Key Question
MI	myocardial infarction
NA	not available
NR	not reported
OR	odds ratio
PICOTS	population, intervention, comparator, outcomes, timing, setting
QOL	quality of life
RCT	randomized controlled trial
ROB	risk of bias
RR	risk ratio
SMI	serious mental illness
SOE	strength of evidence
TEP	Technical Expert Panel

Appendix A. Exact Search Strings

PubMed® Search Strategy (July 20, 2012)

Table A-1. PubMed search strings for KQ 1

Set #	Terms
#1	Schizophrenia[tiab] OR schizophrenia[mesh] OR bipolar disorder[mesh:noexp] OR "bipolar disorder"[tiab] OR "psychotic disorders"[tiab] OR schizoaffective[tiab] OR mania[ti] OR manic[ti] OR "bipolar affective disorder"[tiab] OR "serious mental illness"[tiab] OR "severe mental illness"[tiab] OR "severe psychiatric illness"[tiab] OR ("depressive disorder"[mesh] AND psychotic[tiab]) OR "affective disorders, psychotic"[mesh] OR "psychotic disorders"[mesh]
#2	overweight[mesh] OR overweight[tiab] OR obesity[mesh] OR obesity[tiab] OR obese[tiab] OR weight[tiab] OR Body weights and measures[mesh] OR "body mass index"[tw] OR bmi[tw]
#3	chlorpromazine[MeSH] OR chlorpromazine[tw] OR thorazine[tw] OR fluphenazine[MeSH] OR fluphenazine[tw] OR haloperidol[MeSH] OR haloperidol[tw] OR haldol[tw] OR iloperidone[Supplementary Concept] OR iloperidone[tw] OR fanapt[tw] OR loxapine[MeSH] OR loxapine[tw] OR loxitane[tw] OR molindone[MeSH] OR molindone[tw] OR moban[tw] OR chlorpromazine[MeSH] OR chlorpromazine[tw] OR thorazine[tw] OR perphenazine[MeSH] OR perphenazine[tw] OR pimozide[MeSH] OR pimozide[tw] OR orap[tw] OR thioridazine[MeSH] OR thioridazine[tw] OR thiothixene[MeSH] OR thiothixene[tw] OR navane[tw] OR trifluoperazine[MeSH] OR trifluoperazine[tw] OR stelazine[tw] OR clozapine[MeSH] OR clozapine[tw] OR clozaril[tw] OR risperidone[MeSH] OR risperidone[tw] OR risperidal[tw] OR olanzapine[Supplementary Concept] OR olanzapine[tw] OR zyprexa[tw] OR quetiapine[Supplementary Concept] OR quetiapine[tw] OR seroquel[tw] OR ziprasidone[Supplementary Concept] OR ziprasidone[tw] OR geodon[tw] OR aripiprazole[Supplementary Concept] OR aripiprazole[tw] OR abilify[tw] OR 9-hydroxy-risperidone[Supplementary Concept] OR "9-hydroxy-risperidone"[tw] OR paliperidone[tw] OR invega[tw] OR antipsychotic agents[mh] OR antipsychotic agents[pharmacological action] OR antipsychotic[tiab] OR antipsychotics[tiab]
#4	#1 AND (#2 OR #3)
#5	orlistat[Supplementary Concept] OR orlistat[tw] OR topiramate[Supplementary Concept] OR topiramate[tw] OR metformin[MeSH] OR metformin[tw] OR amantadine[MeSH] OR amantadine[tw] OR "Appetite Depressants"[Mesh] OR "Appetite Depressants" [Pharmacological Action] OR "Anti-Obesity Agents"[Mesh] OR "Anti-Obesity Agents" [Pharmacological Action]
#6	"Nutrition Therapy"[Mesh] OR "Exercise"[Mesh] OR "Exercise Therapy"[Mesh] OR "Exercise Movement Techniques"[Mesh] OR "diet therapy"[mesh] OR exercise[tiab] OR "physical activity"[tiab] OR diet[tiab] OR diets[tiab] OR "weight management"[tiab] OR "Behavior Therapy"[Mesh] OR health education[mesh] OR health promotion[mesh] OR counsel*[tiab] OR counseling[mesh] OR "disease management"[mesh] OR "cognitive behavioral therapy"[tiab] OR "lifestyle modification"[tiab] OR ("life style"[mesh] AND modification[tiab]) OR "Patient Compliance"[Mesh] OR adher*[tiab] OR "self-monitoring"[tiab] OR "Recurrence/prevention and control"[Mesh] OR "relapse prevention"[tiab] OR "skills training"[tiab] OR "motivational interviewing"[tiab] OR educat*[tiab]
#7	social support[mesh] OR family[tiab] OR peer[tiab]
#8	Drug substitution[mesh] OR substitut*[tw] switch[tiab] OR switched[tiab] OR switching[tiab] OR change[tiab] OR changed[tiab] OR changing[tiab] OR replace[tiab] OR replaced[tiab] OR replacing[tiab] OR replacement[tiab] OR abandon*[tiab]
#9	#5 OR #6 OR #7 OR #8
#10	(randomized controlled trial[pt] OR controlled clinical trial[pt] OR randomized[tiab] OR randomised[tiab] OR randomization[tiab] OR randomisation[tiab] OR placebo[tiab] OR randomly[tiab] OR trial[tiab] OR groups[tiab]) NOT (animals[mh] NOT humans[mh]) NOT (Editorial[ptyp] OR Letter[ptyp] OR Case Reports[ptyp] OR Comment[ptyp])
#11	#4 AND #9 AND #10, Limits: English

Table A-2. PubMed search strings for KQ 2

Set #	Terms
#1	Schizophrenia[tiab] OR schizophrenia[mesh] OR bipolar disorder[mesh:noexp] OR "bipolar disorder"[tiab] OR "psychotic disorders"[tiab] OR schizoaffective[tiab] OR mania[ti] OR manic[ti] OR "bipolar affective disorder"[tiab] OR "serious mental illness"[tiab] OR "severe mental illness"[tiab] OR "severe psychiatric illness"[tiab] OR ("depressive disorder"[mesh] AND psychotic[tiab]) OR "affective disorders, psychotic"[mesh] OR "psychotic disorders"[mesh]
#2	Diabetes mellitus[mesh] OR diabetes[tiab]
#3	chlorpromazine[MeSH] OR chlorpromazine[tw] OR thorazine[tw] OR fluphenazine[MeSH] OR fluphenazine[tw] OR haloperidol[MeSH] OR haloperidol[tw] OR haldol[tw] OR iloperidone[Supplementary Concept] OR iloperidone[tw] OR fanapt[tw] OR loxapine[MeSH] OR loxapine[tw] OR loxitane[tw] OR molindone[MeSH] OR molindone[tw] OR moban[tw] OR chlorpromazine[MeSH] OR chlorpromazine[tw] OR thorazine[tw] OR perphenazine[MeSH] OR perphenazine[tw] OR pimozide[MeSH] OR pimozide[tw] OR orap[tw] OR thioridazine[MeSH] OR thioridazine[tw] OR thiothixene[MeSH] OR thiothixene[tw] OR navane[tw] OR trifluoperazine[MeSH] OR trifluoperazine[tw] OR stelazine[tw] OR clozapine[MeSH] OR clozapine[tw] OR clozaril[tw] OR risperidone[MeSH] OR risperidone[tw] OR risperidal[tw] OR olanzapine[Supplementary Concept] OR olanzapine[tw] OR zyprexa[tw] OR quetiapine[Supplementary Concept] OR quetiapine[tw] OR seroquel[tw] OR ziprasidone[Supplementary Concept] OR ziprasidone[tw] OR geodon[tw] OR aripiprazole[Supplementary Concept] OR aripiprazole[tw] OR abilify[tw] OR 9-hydroxy-risperidone[Supplementary Concept] OR "9-hydroxy-risperidone"[tw] OR paliperidone[tw] OR invega[tw] OR antipsychotic agents[mh] OR antipsychotic agents[pharmacological action] OR antipsychotic[tiab] OR antipsychotics[tiab]
#4	#1 AND (#2 OR #3)
#5	"exenatide"[Supplementary Concept] OR Byetta[tiab] OR exenatide[tiab] OR "pramlintide"[Supplementary Concept] OR Symlin[tiab] OR *pramlintide* [tiab] OR "sitagliptin"[Supplementary Concept] OR Januvia[tiab] OR sitagliptin[tiab] OR glargine[supplementary concept] OR Lantus[tiab] OR "insulin glargine"[tiab] OR "saxagliptin"[Supplementary Concept] OR Onglyza[tiab] OR saxagliptin[tiab] OR "miglitol"[Supplementary Concept] OR Glyset[tiab] OR miglitol[tiab] OR "rosiglitazone"[Supplementary Concept] OR Avandia[tiab] OR rosiglitazone[tiab] OR "pioglitazone"[Supplementary Concept] OR Actos[tiab] OR pioglitazone[tiab] OR "repaglinide"[Supplementary Concept] OR Prandin[tiab] OR repaglinide[tiab] OR "nateglinide"[Supplementary Concept] OR Starlix[tiab] OR nateglinide[tiab] OR "glyburide"[MeSH] OR Diabeta[tiab] OR glyburide[tiab] OR "glimepiride"[Supplementary Concept]OR Amaryl[tiab] OR glimepiride[tiab] OR "metformin"[MeSH] OR Glumetza[tiab] OR metformin[tiab] OR Riomet[tiab] OR Fortamet[tiab] OR "BI 1356"[Supplementary Concept] OR Tradjenta[tiab] OR linagliptin[tiab] OR "liraglutide"[Supplementary Concept]OR Victoza[tiab] OR liraglutide[tiab] OR "colesevelam"[Supplementary Concept] OR WelChol[tiab] OR colesevelam[tiab] OR "bromocriptine"[MeSH] OR Cycloset[tiab] OR bromocriptine[tiab] OR Parlodel[tiab] OR "Hypoglycemic Agents"[Mesh] OR "Hypoglycemic Agents" [Pharmacological Action]
#6	"Diabetes Mellitus/prevention and control"[Mesh] OR "diabetes management"[tiab] OR "Behavior Therapy"[Mesh] OR health education[mesh] OR health promotion[mesh] OR counsel*[tiab] OR counseling[mesh] OR "disease management"[mesh] OR "cognitive behavioral therapy"[tiab] OR "lifestyle modification"[tiab] OR ("life style"[mesh] AND modification[tiab]) OR "Patient Compliance"[Mesh] OR adher*[tiab] OR "self-monitoring"[tiab] OR "Recurrence/prevention and control"[Mesh] OR "relapse prevention"[tiab] OR "skills training"[tiab] OR "motivational interviewing"[tiab] OR educat*[tiab]
#7	social support[mesh] OR family[tiab] OR peer[tiab]
#8	Drug substitution[mesh] OR substitut*[tw] switch[tiab] OR switched[tiab] OR switching[tiab] OR change[tiab] OR changed[tiab] OR changing[tiab] OR replace[tiab] OR replaced[tiab] OR replacing[tiab] OR replacement[tiab] OR abandon*[tiab]
#9	#5 OR #6 OR #7 OR #8
#10	#4 AND #9
#11	(randomized controlled trial[pt] OR controlled clinical trial[pt] OR randomized[tiab] OR randomised[tiab] OR randomization[tiab] OR randomisation[tiab] OR placebo[tiab] OR randomly[tiab] OR trial[tiab] OR groups[tiab]) NOT (animals[mh] NOT humans[mh]) NOT (Editorial[ptyp] OR Letter[ptyp] OR Case Reports[ptyp] OR Comment[ptyp])
#12	#10 AND #11, Limits: English

Table A-3. PubMed search strings for KQ 3

Set #	Terms
#1	Schizophrenia[tiab] OR schizophrenia[mesh] OR bipolar disorder[mesh:noexp] OR "bipolar disorder"[tiab] OR "psychotic disorders"[tiab] OR schizoaffective[tiab] OR mania[ti] OR manic[ti] OR "bipolar affective disorder"[tiab] OR "serious mental illness"[tiab] OR "severe mental illness"[tiab] OR "severe psychiatric illness"[tiab] OR ("depressive disorder"[mesh] AND psychotic[tiab]) OR "affective disorders, psychotic"[mesh] OR "psychotic disorders"[mesh]
#2	"Dyslipidemias"[Mesh] OR "Hyperlipidemias"[Mesh] OR dyslipidemia[tiab] OR dyslipidemias[tiab] OR hyperlipidemia[tiab] OR hyperlipidemias[tiab]
#3	chlorpromazine[MeSH] OR chlorpromazine[tw] OR thorazine[tw] OR fluphenazine[MeSH] OR fluphenazine[tw] OR haloperidol[MeSH] OR haloperidol[tw] OR haldol[tw] OR iloperidone[Supplementary Concept] OR iloperidone[tw] OR fanapt[tw] OR loxapine[MeSH] OR loxapine[tw] OR loxitane[tw] OR molindone[MeSH] OR molindone[tw] OR moban[tw] OR chlorpromazine[MeSH] OR chlorpromazine[tw] OR thorazine[tw] OR perphenazine[MeSH] OR perphenazine[tw] OR pimozide[MeSH] OR pimozide[tw] OR orap[tw] OR thioridazine[MeSH] OR thioridazine[tw] OR thiothixene[MeSH] OR thiothixene[tw] OR navane[tw] OR trifluoperazine[MeSH] OR trifluoperazine[tw] OR stelazine[tw] OR clozapine[MeSH] OR clozapine[tw] OR clozaril[tw] OR risperidone[MeSH] OR risperidone[tw] OR risperidal[tw] OR olanzapine[Supplementary Concept] OR olanzapine[tw] OR zyprexa[tw] OR quetiapine[Supplementary Concept] OR quetiapine[tw] OR seroquel[tw] OR ziprasidone[Supplementary Concept] OR ziprasidone[tw] OR geodon[tw] OR aripiprazole[Supplementary Concept] OR aripiprazole[tw] OR abilify[tw] OR 9-hydroxy-risperidone[Supplementary Concept] OR "9-hydroxy-risperidone"[tw] OR paliperidone[tw] OR invega[tw] OR antipsychotic agents[mh] OR antipsychotic agents[pharmacological action] OR antipsychotic[tiab] OR antipsychotics[tiab]
#4	#1 AND (#2 OR #3)
#5	"Hypolipidemic Agents"[Mesh] OR "Hypolipidemic Agents" [Pharmacological Action] OR "Hydroxymethylglutaryl-CoA Reductase Inhibitors"[Mesh] OR "Hydroxymethylglutaryl-CoA Reductase Inhibitors" [Pharmacological Action] OR statins[tiab] OR statin[tiab] OR "Simvastatin"[Mesh] OR simvastatin[tiab] OR "Lovastatin"[Mesh] OR lovastatin[tiab] OR "atorvastatin" [Supplementary Concept] OR atorvastatin[tiab] OR "Pravastatin"[Mesh] OR pravastatin[tiab] OR "fluvastatin" [Supplementary Concept] OR fluvastatin[tiab] OR "pitavastatin" [Supplementary Concept] OR pitavastatin[tiab] OR "ezetimibe" [Supplementary Concept] OR Ezetimibe[tiab] OR "Niacin"[Mesh] OR niacin[tiab] OR "Fenofibrate"[Mesh] OR fenofibrate[tiab] OR "Fibric Acids"[Mesh] OR "fibric acid"[tiab] OR "fibric acids"[tiab] OR fibrates[tiab] OR fibrate[tiab] OR "Gemfibrozil"[Mesh] OR gemfibrozil[tiab] OR "Colestipol"[Mesh] OR "Cholestyramine Resin"[Mesh] OR Colestipol[tiab] OR Cholestyramine[tiab] OR "colesevelam" [Supplementary Concept] OR colesevelam[tiab]
#6	"Nutrition Therapy"[Mesh] OR "Exercise"[Mesh] OR "Exercise Therapy"[Mesh] OR "Exercise Movement Techniques"[Mesh] OR "diet therapy"[mesh] OR exercise[tiab] OR "physical activity"[tiab] OR diet[tiab] OR diets[tiab] OR "weight management"[tiab] OR "Behavior Therapy"[Mesh] OR health education[mesh] OR health promotion[mesh] OR counsel*[tiab] OR counseling[mesh] OR "disease management"[mesh] OR "cognitive behavioral therapy"[tiab] OR "lifestyle modification"[tiab] OR ("life style"[mesh] AND modification[tiab]) OR "Patient Compliance"[Mesh] OR adher*[tiab] OR "self-monitoring"[tiab] OR "Recurrence/prevention and control"[Mesh] OR "relapse prevention"[tiab] OR "skills training"[tiab] OR "motivational interviewing"[tiab] OR educat*[tiab]
#7	social support[mesh] OR family[tiab] OR peer[tiab]
#8	Drug substitution[mesh] OR substitut*[tw] switch[tiab] OR switched[tiab] OR switching[tiab] OR change[tiab] OR changed[tiab] OR changing[tiab] OR replace[tiab] OR replaced[tiab] OR replacing[tiab] OR replacement[tiab] OR abandon*[tiab]
#9	#5 OR #6 OR #7 OR #8
#10	(randomized controlled trial[pt] OR controlled clinical trial[pt] OR randomized[tiab] OR randomised[tiab] OR randomization[tiab] OR randomisation[tiab] OR placebo[tiab] OR randomly[tiab] OR trial[tiab] OR groups[tiab]) NOT (animals[mh] NOT humans[mh]) NOT (Editorial[ptyp] OR Letter[ptyp] OR Case Reports[ptyp] OR Comment[ptyp])
#11	#4 AND #9 AND #10, Limits: English

Table A-4. PubMed search strings for KQ 4

Set #	Terms
#1	Schizophrenia[tiab] OR schizophrenia[mesh] OR bipolar disorder[mesh:noexp] OR "bipolar disorder"[tiab] OR "psychotic disorders"[tiab] OR schizoaffective[tiab] OR mania[ti] OR manic[ti] OR "bipolar affective disorder"[tiab] OR "serious mental illness"[tiab] OR "severe mental illness"[tiab] OR "severe psychiatric illness"[tiab] OR ("depressive disorder"[mesh] AND psychotic[tiab]) OR "affective disorders, psychotic"[mesh] OR "psychotic disorders"[mesh]
#2	"Cardiovascular Diseases"[Mesh] OR "Hyperlipidemias"[Mesh] OR hypertension[tiab] OR ((cardiovascular[tiab] OR heart[tiab] OR coronary[tiab]) AND (disease[tiab] OR diseases[tiab] OR risk[tiab]))
#3	chlorpromazine[MeSH] OR chlorpromazine[tw] OR thorazine[tw] OR fluphenazine[MeSH] OR fluphenazine[tw] OR haloperidol[MeSH] OR haloperidol[tw] OR haldol[tw] OR iloperidone[Supplementary Concept] OR iloperidone[tw] OR fanapt[tw] OR loxapine[MeSH] OR loxapine[tw] OR loxitane[tw] OR molindone[MeSH] OR molindone[tw] OR moban[tw] OR chlorpromazine[MeSH] OR chlorpromazine[tw] OR thorazine[tw] OR perphenazine[MeSH] OR perphenazine[tw] OR pimozide[MeSH] OR pimozide[tw] OR orap[tw] OR thioridazine[MeSH] OR thioridazine[tw] OR thiothixene[MeSH] OR thiothixene[tw] OR navane[tw] OR trifluoperazine[MeSH] OR trifluoperazine[tw] OR stelazine[tw] OR clozapine[MeSH] OR clozapine[tw] OR clozaril[tw] OR risperidone[MeSH] OR risperidone[tw] OR risperidal[tw] OR olanzapine[Supplementary Concept] OR olanzapine[tw] OR zyprexa[tw] OR quetiapine[Supplementary Concept] OR quetiapine[tw] OR seroquel[tw] OR ziprasidone[Supplementary Concept] OR ziprasidone[tw] OR geodon[tw] OR aripiprazole[Supplementary Concept] OR aripiprazole[tw] OR abilify[tw] OR 9-hydroxy-risperidone[Supplementary Concept] OR "9-hydroxy-risperidone"[tw] OR paliperidone[tw] OR invega[tw] OR antipsychotic agents[mh] OR antipsychotic agents[pharmacological action] OR antipsychotic[tiab] OR antipsychotics[tiab]
#4	#1 AND (#2 OR #3)

Set #	Terms
#5	atorvastatin[Supplementary Concept] OR cholestyramine resin[MeSH] OR colesevelam[Supplementary Concept] colestipol[MeSH] OR ezetimibe[Supplementary Concept] OR fenofibrate[MeSH] OR fluvastatin[Supplementary Concept] OR lovastatin[MeSH] OR pitavastatin[Supplementary Concept] OR pravastatin[MeSH] OR rosuvastatin[Supplementary Concept] OR simvastatin[MeSH] OR acebutolol[Mesh] OR aliskiren[Supplementary Concept] OR amiloride[Mesh] OR amlodipine[Mesh] OR atenolol[Mesh] OR "2-ethoxy-1-((2'-(5-oxo-2,5-dihydro-1,2,4-oxadiazol-3-yl)-biphenyl-4-yl)methyl)-1H-benzimidazole-7-carboxylic acid"[Supplementary Concept] OR benazepril[Supplementary Concept] OR betaxolol[Mesh] OR bisoprolol[Mesh] OR candesartan[Supplementary Concept] OR carvedilol[Supplementary Concept] OR chlorothiazide[Mesh] OR chlorthalidone[Mesh] OR clonidine[Mesh] OR diltiazem[Mesh] OR irbesartan[Supplementary Concept] OR isradipine[Mesh] OR labetalol[Mesh] OR lisinopril[Mesh] OR losartan[Mesh] OR metolazone[Mesh] OR metoprolol[Mesh] OR moexipril[Supplementary Concept] OR nebivolol[Supplementary Concept] OR nicardipine[Mesh] OR nifedipine[Mesh] OR nisoldipine[Mesh] OR olmesartan[Supplementary Concept] OR penbutolol[Mesh] OR perindopril[Mesh] OR pindolol[Mesh] OR prazosin[Mesh] OR propranolol[Mesh] OR quinapril[Supplementary Concept] OR ramipril[Mesh] OR telmisartan[Supplementary Concept] OR torsemide[Supplementary Concept] OR trandolapril[Supplementary Concept] OR valsartan[Supplementary Concept] OR verapamil[Mesh] OR Lipitor[tiab] OR atorvastatin[tiab] OR Caduet[tiab] OR Prevalite[tiab] OR cholestyramine[tiab] OR Questran[tiab] OR WelChol[tiab] OR colesevelam[tiab] OR Colestid[tiab] OR colestipol[tiab] OR Zetia[tiab] OR ezetimibe[tiab] OR Tricor[tiab] OR fenofibrate[tiab] OR Lescol[tiab] OR fluvastatin[tiab] OR Mevacor[tiab] OR lovastatin[tiab] OR Livalo[tiab] OR pitavastatin[tiab] OR Pravachol[tiab] OR pravastatin[tiab] OR Crestor[tiab] OR rosuvastatin[tiab] OR Zocor[tiab] OR simvastatin[tiab] OR Sectral[tiab] OR Acebutolol[tiab] OR Tekturna[tiab] OR Aliskiren[tiab] OR Tekamlo[tiab] OR Valturna[tiab] OR Midimor[tiab] OR Amiloride[tiab] OR Norvasc[tiab] OR Amlodipine[tiab] OR Caduet[tiab] OR Lotrel[tiab] OR Tenormin[tiab] OR Atenolol[tiab] OR Tenoretic[tiab] OR Edarbi[tiab] OR Azilsartan[tiab] OR Lotensin[tiab] OR Benazepril[tiab] OR Kerlone[tiab] OR Betaxolol[tiab] OR Zebeta[tiab] OR Bisoprolol[tiab] OR Atacand[tiab] OR Candesartan[tiab] OR Coreg[tiab] OR Carvedilol[tiab] OR Diuril[tiab] OR Chlorothiazide[tiab] OR Thalitone[tiab] OR Chlorthalidone[tiab] OR Clorpres[tiab] OR Catapres[tiab] OR Clonidine[tiab] OR Cardizem[tiab] OR diltiazem[tiab] OR Cartia[tiab] OR Dilacor[tiab] OR Dilt[tiab] OR Diltia[tiab] OR Matzim[tiab] OR Taztia[tiab] OR Tiamate[tiab] OR Tiazac[tiab] OR Avapro[tiab] OR irbesartan[tiab] OR Dynacirc[tiab] OR isradipine[tiab] OR Trandate[tiab] OR labetalol[tiab] OR Prinivil[tiab] OR lisinopril[tiab] OR Zestril[tiab] OR Cozaar[tiab] OR losartan[tiab] OR Zaroxloyn[tiab] OR metolazone[tiab] OR Lopressor[tiab] OR metoprolol[tiab] OR Toprol[tiab] OR Univasc[tiab] OR moexipril[tiab] OR Corgard[tiab] OR nadalol[tiab] OR Bystolic[tiab] OR nebivolol[tiab] OR Cardene[tiab] OR nicardipine[tiab] OR Procardia[tiab] OR nifedipine[tiab] OR Sular[tiab] OR nisoldipine[tiab] OR Benicar[tiab] OR olmesartan[tiab] OR Levitol[tiab] OR penbutolol[tiab] OR Aceon[tiab] OR perindopril[tiab] OR Pindolol[tiab] OR pindolol[tiab] OR Minipress[tiab] OR prazosin[tiab] OR Inderal[tiab] OR propranolol[tiab] OR Accupril[tiab] OR quinapril[tiab] OR Altace[tiab] OR ramipril[tiab] OR Micardis[tiab] OR telmisartan[tiab] OR Demadex[tiab] OR torsemide[tiab] OR Mavik[tiab] OR trandolapril[tiab] OR Diovan[tiab] OR valsartan[tiab] OR Calan[tiab] OR verapamil[tiab] OR Covera[tiab] OR Isoptin[tiab] OR Verelan[tiab] OR "Antihypertensive Agents"[Mesh] OR "Antihypertensive Agents" [Pharmacological Action] OR "Hypolipidemic Agents"[Mesh] OR "Nicotinic Agonists"[Mesh] OR "Nicotinic Agonists" [Pharmacological Action] OR "Cardiovascular Agents"[Mesh] OR "Cardiovascular Agents" [Pharmacological Action] OR "Heparin"[Mesh] OR "Heparin, Low-Molecular-Weight"[Mesh] OR "Warfarin"[Mesh] OR heparin[tiab] OR warfarin[tiab] OR bupropion[tiab] OR "Bupropion"[Mesh]
#6	Smoking cessation[mesh] OR smoking[tiab] OR tobacco[tiab] OR "Nutrition Therapy"[Mesh] OR "Exercise"[Mesh] OR "Exercise Therapy"[Mesh] OR "Exercise Movement Techniques"[Mesh] OR diet therapy[mesh] OR exercise[tiab] OR "physical activity"[tiab] OR diet[tiab] OR diets[tiab] OR "Behavior Therapy"[Mesh] OR health education[mesh] OR health promotion[mesh] OR counsel*[tiab] OR counseling[mesh] OR "disease management"[mesh] OR "cognitive behavioral therapy"[tiab] OR "lifestyle modification"[tiab] OR ("life style"[mesh] AND modification[tiab]) OR "Patient Compliance"[Mesh] OR adher*[tiab] OR "self-monitoring"[tiab] OR "Recurrence/prevention and control"[Mesh] OR "relapse prevention"[tiab] OR "skills training"[tiab] OR "motivational interviewing"[tiab] OR educat*[tiab]
#7	social support[mesh] OR family[tiab] OR peer[tiab]
#8	Drug substitution[mesh] OR substitut*[tw] switch[tiab] OR switched[tiab] OR switching[tiab] OR change[tiab] OR changed[tiab] OR changing[tiab] OR replace[tiab] OR replaced[tiab] OR replacing[tiab] OR replacement[tiab] OR abandon*[tiab]
#9	#5 OR #6 OR #7 OR #8

Set #	Terms
#10	(randomized controlled trial[pt] OR controlled clinical trial[pt] OR randomized[tiab] OR randomised[tiab] OR randomization[tiab] OR randomisation[tiab] OR placebo[tiab] OR randomly[tiab] OR trial[tiab] OR groups[tiab]) NOT (animals[mh] NOT humans[mh]) NOT (Editorial[ptyp] OR Letter[ptyp] OR Case Reports[ptyp] OR Comment[ptyp])
#11	#4 AND #9 AND #10, Limits: English

Embase® Search Strategy (July 20, 2012)

Platform: Embase.com

Table A-5. Embase search strings for KQ 1

Set #	Terms
#1	'schizophrenia'/exp OR 'bipolar disorder'/exp OR 'affective psychosis'/exp OR 'depressive psychosis'/exp OR 'manic depressive psychosis'/exp OR schizophrenia:ab,ti OR 'bipolar disorder':ab,ti OR 'psychotic disorders':ab,ti OR schizoaffective:ab,ti OR mania:ti OR manic:ti OR 'bipolar affective disorder':ab,ti OR 'serious mental illness':ab,ti OR 'severe mental illness':ab,ti OR 'severe psychiatric illness':ab,ti
#2	'obesity'/exp OR 'body weight'/exp OR 'body mass'/exp OR overweight:ab,ti OR obesity:ab,ti OR obese:ab,ti OR weight:ab,ti OR "body mass index":ab,ti OR bmi:ab,ti
#3	'chlorpromazine'/exp OR chlorpromazine:ab,ti OR thorazine:ab,ti OR 'fluphenazine'/exp OR fluphenazine:ab,ti OR 'haloperidol'/exp OR haloperidol:ab,ti OR haldol:ab,ti OR 'iloperidone'/exp OR iloperidone:ab,ti OR fanapt:ab,ti OR 'loxapine'/exp OR loxapine:ab,ti OR loxitane:ab,ti OR 'molindone'/exp OR molindone:ab,ti OR moban:ab,ti OR 'chlorpromazine'/exp OR chlorpromazine:ab,ti OR thorazine:ab,ti OR 'perphenazine'/exp OR perphenazine:ab,ti OR 'pimozide'/exp OR pimozide:ab,ti OR orap:ab,ti OR 'thioridazine'/exp OR thioridazine:ab,ti OR 'tiotixene'/exp OR thiothixene:ab,ti OR navane:ab,ti OR 'trifluoperazine'/exp OR trifluoperazine:ab,ti OR stelazine:ab,ti OR 'clozapine'/exp OR clozapine:ab,ti OR clozaril:ab,ti OR 'risperidone'/exp OR risperidone:ab,ti OR risperidal:ab,ti OR 'olanzapine'/exp OR olanzapine:ab,ti OR zyprexa:ab,ti OR 'quetiapine'/exp OR quetiapine:ab,ti OR seroquel:ab,ti OR 'ziprasidone'/exp OR ziprasidone:ab,ti OR geodon:ab,ti OR 'aripiprazole'/exp OR aripiprazole:ab,ti OR abilify:ab,ti OR "9-hydroxy-risperidone":ab,ti OR paliperidone:ab,ti OR invega:ab,ti OR 'neuroleptic agent'/exp OR antipsychotic:ab,ti OR antipsychotics:ab,ti
#4	#1 AND (#2 OR #3)
#5	'tetrahydrolipstatin'/exp OR orlistat:ab,ti OR 'topiramate'/exp OR topiramate:ab,ti OR 'metformin'/exp OR metformin:ab,ti OR 'amantadine'/exp OR amantadine:ab,ti OR 'anorexigenic agent'/exp OR 'antiobesity agent'/exp
#6	'diet therapy'/exp OR 'exercise'/exp OR 'kinesiotherapy'/exp OR 'low calory diet'/exp OR exercise:ab,ti OR "physical activity":ab,ti OR diet:ab,ti OR diets:ab,ti OR 'weight reduction'/exp OR "weight management":ab,ti OR 'behavior therapy'/exp OR 'cognitive therapy'/exp OR 'health education' OR counsel*:ab,ti OR 'counseling'/exp OR 'disease management'/exp OR 'lifestyle modification'/exp OR "lifestyle modification":ab,ti OR 'patient compliance'/exp OR "cognitive behavioral therapy":ab,ti OR adher*:ab,ti OR "self-monitoring":ab,ti OR 'recurrent disease'/exp/dm_pc OR "relapse prevention":ab,ti OR "skills training":ab,ti OR "motivational interviewing":ab,ti OR educat*:ab,ti
#7	'social support'/exp OR family:ab,ti OR peer:ab,ti
#8	'drug substitution'/exp OR substitut*:ab,ti switch:ab,ti OR switched:ab,ti OR switching:ab,ti OR change:ab,ti OR changed:ab,ti OR changing:ab,ti OR replace:ab,ti OR replaced:ab,ti OR replacing:ab,ti OR replacement:ab,ti OR abandon*:ab,ti
#9	#5 OR #6 OR #7 OR #8
#10	'controlled clinical trial'/exp OR randomized:ab,ti OR randomised:ab,ti OR randomization:ab,ti OR randomisation:ab,ti OR placebo:ab,ti OR randomly:ab,ti OR trial:ab,ti OR groups:ab,ti NOT ('case report'/exp OR 'case study'/exp OR 'editorial'/exp OR 'letter'/exp OR 'note'/exp)
#11	#4 AND #9 AND #10
#12	#11 AND [embase]/lim NOT [medline]/lim, Limits: English, Human

Table A-6. Embase search strings for KQ 2

Set #	Terms
#1	'schizophrenia'/exp OR 'bipolar disorder'/exp OR 'affective psychosis'/exp OR 'depressive psychosis'/exp OR 'manic depressive psychosis'/exp OR schizophrenia:ab,ti OR 'bipolar disorder':ab,ti OR 'psychotic disorders':ab,ti OR schizoaffective:ab,ti OR mania:ti OR manic:ti OR 'bipolar affective disorder':ab,ti OR 'serious mental illness':ab,ti OR 'severe mental illness':ab,ti OR 'severe psychiatric illness':ab,ti
#2	'diabetes mellitus'/exp OR diabetes:ab,ti
#3	'chlorpromazine'/exp OR chlorpromazine:ab,ti OR thorazine:ab,ti OR 'fluphenazine'/exp OR fluphenazine:ab,ti OR 'haloperidol'/exp OR haloperidol:ab,ti OR haldol:ab,ti OR 'iloperidone'/exp OR iloperidone:ab,ti OR fanapt:ab,ti OR 'loxapine'/exp OR loxapine:ab,ti OR loxitane:ab,ti OR 'molindone'/exp OR molindone:ab,ti OR moban:ab,ti OR 'chlorpromazine'/exp OR chlorpromazine:ab,ti OR thorazine:ab,ti OR 'perphenazine'/exp OR perphenazine:ab,ti OR 'pimozide'/exp OR pimozide:ab,ti OR orap:ab,ti OR 'thioridazine'/exp OR thioridazine:ab,ti OR 'tiotixene'/exp OR thiothixene:ab,ti OR navane:ab,ti OR 'trifluoperazine'/exp OR trifluoperazine:ab,ti OR stelazine:ab,ti OR 'clozapine'/exp OR clozapine:ab,ti OR clozaril:ab,ti OR 'risperidone'/exp OR risperidone:ab,ti OR risperidal:ab,ti OR 'olanzapine'/exp OR olanzapine:ab,ti OR zyprexa:ab,ti OR 'quetiapine'/exp OR quetiapine:ab,ti OR seroquel:ab,ti OR 'ziprasidone'/exp OR ziprasidone:ab,ti OR geodon:ab,ti OR 'aripiprazole'/exp OR aripiprazole:ab,ti OR abilify:ab,ti OR "9-hydroxy-risperidone":ab,ti OR paliperidone:ab,ti OR invega:ab,ti OR 'neuroleptic agent'/exp OR antipsychotic:ab,ti OR antipsychotics:ab,ti
#4	#1 AND (#2 OR #3)
#5	'exendin 4'/exp OR Byetta:ab,ti OR exenatide:ab,ti OR 'pramlintide'/exp OR Symlin:ab,ti OR pramlintide:ab,ti OR 'sitagliptin'/exp OR Januvia:ab,ti OR sitagliptin:ab,ti OR 'insulin glargine'/exp OR Lantus:ab,ti OR "insulin glargine":ab,ti OR 'saxagliptin'/exp OR Onglyza:ab,ti OR saxagliptin:ab,ti OR 'miglitol'/exp OR Glyset:ab,ti OR miglitol:ab,ti OR 'rosiglitazone'/exp OR Avandia:ab,ti OR rosiglitazone:ab,ti OR 'pioglitazone'/exp OR Actos:ab,ti OR pioglitazone:ab,ti OR 'repaglinide'/exp OR Prandin:ab,ti OR repaglinide:ab,ti OR 'nateglinide'/exp OR Starlix:ab,ti OR nateglinide:ab,ti OR 'glibenclamide'/exp OR Diabeta:ab,ti OR glyburide:ab,ti OR 'glimepiride'/exp OR Amaryl:ab,ti OR glimepiride:ab,ti OR 'metformin'/exp OR Glumetza:ab,ti OR metformin:ab,ti OR Riomet:ab,ti OR Fortamet:ab,ti OR 'linagliptin'/exp OR Tradjenta:ab,ti OR linagliptin:ab,ti OR 'liraglutide'/exp OR Victoza:ab,ti OR liraglutide:ab,ti OR 'colesevelam'/exp OR WelChol:ab,ti OR colesevelam:ab,ti OR 'bromocriptine'/exp OR Cycloset:ab,ti OR bromocriptine:ab,ti OR Parlodel:ab,ti OR 'antidiabetic agent'/exp
#6	'diabetes mellitus'/exp/dm_dm OR "diabetes management":ab,ti OR 'diet therapy'/exp OR 'exercise'/exp OR 'kinesiotherapy'/exp OR 'low calory diet'/exp OR exercise:ab,ti OR "physical activity":ab,ti OR diet:ab,ti OR diets:ab,ti OR 'weight reduction'/exp OR "weight management":ab,ti OR 'behavior therapy'/exp OR 'cognitive therapy'/exp OR 'health education' OR counsel*:ab,ti OR 'counseling'/exp OR 'disease management'/exp OR 'lifestyle modification'/exp OR "lifestyle modification":ab,ti OR 'patient compliance'/exp OR "cognitive behavioral therapy":ab,ti OR adher*:ab,ti OR "self-monitoring":ab,ti OR 'recurrent disease'/exp/dm_pc OR "relapse prevention":ab,ti OR "skills training":ab,ti OR "motivational interviewing":ab,ti OR educat*:ab,ti
#7	'social support'/exp OR family:ab,ti OR peer:ab,ti
#8	'drug substitution'/exp OR substitut*:ab,ti switch:ab,ti OR switched:ab,ti OR switching:ab,ti OR change:ab,ti OR changed:ab,ti OR changing:ab,ti OR replace:ab,ti OR replaced:ab,ti OR replacing:ab,ti OR replacement:ab,ti OR abandon*:ab,ti
#9	#5 OR #6 OR #7 OR #8
#10	'controlled clinical trial'/exp OR randomized:ab,ti OR randomised:ab,ti OR randomization:ab,ti OR randomisation:ab,ti OR placebo:ab,ti OR randomly:ab,ti OR trial:ab,ti OR groups:ab,ti NOT ('case report'/exp OR 'case study'/exp OR 'editorial'/exp OR 'letter'/exp OR 'note'/exp)
#11	#4 AND #9 AND #10
#12	#11 AND [embase]/lim NOT [medline]/lim, Limits: English, Human

Table A-7. Embase search strings for KQ 3

Set #	Terms
#1	'schizophrenia'/exp OR 'bipolar disorder'/exp OR 'affective psychosis'/exp OR 'depressive psychosis'/exp OR 'manic depressive psychosis'/exp OR schizophrenia:ab,ti OR 'bipolar disorder':ab,ti OR 'psychotic disorders':ab,ti OR schizoaffective:ab,ti OR mania:ti OR manic:ti OR 'bipolar affective disorder':ab,ti OR 'serious mental illness':ab,ti OR 'severe mental illness':ab,ti OR 'severe psychiatric illness':ab,ti
#2	'dyslipidemia'/exp OR 'hyperlipidemia'/exp OR dyslipidemia:ab,ti OR dyslipidemias:ab,ti OR hyperlipidemia:ab,ti OR hyperlipidemias:ab,ti
#3	'chlorpromazine'/exp OR chlorpromazine:ab,ti OR thorazine:ab,ti OR 'fluphenazine'/exp OR fluphenazine:ab,ti OR 'haloperidol'/exp OR haloperidol:ab,ti OR haldol:ab,ti OR 'iloperidone'/exp OR iloperidone:ab,ti OR fanapt:ab,ti OR 'loxapine'/exp OR loxapine:ab,ti OR loxitane:ab,ti OR 'molindone'/exp OR molindone:ab,ti OR moban:ab,ti OR 'chlorpromazine'/exp OR chlorpromazine:ab,ti OR thorazine:ab,ti OR 'perphenazine'/exp OR perphenazine:ab,ti OR 'pimozide'/exp OR pimozide:ab,ti OR orap:ab,ti OR 'thioridazine'/exp OR thioridazine:ab,ti OR 'tiotixene'/exp OR thiothixene:ab,ti OR navane:ab,ti OR 'trifluoperazine'/exp OR trifluoperazine:ab,ti OR stelazine:ab,ti OR 'clozapine'/exp OR clozapine:ab,ti OR clozaril:ab,ti OR 'risperidone'/exp OR risperidone:ab,ti OR risperidal:ab,ti OR 'olanzapine'/exp OR olanzapine:ab,ti OR zyprexa:ab,ti OR 'quetiapine'/exp OR quetiapine:ab,ti OR seroquel:ab,ti OR 'ziprasidone'/exp OR ziprasidone:ab,ti OR geodon:ab,ti OR 'aripiprazole'/exp OR aripiprazole:ab,ti OR abilify:ab,ti OR "9-hydroxy-risperidone":ab,ti OR paliperidone:ab,ti OR invega:ab,ti OR 'neuroleptic agent'/exp OR antipsychotic:ab,ti OR antipsychotics:ab,ti
#4	#1 AND (#2 OR #3)
#5	'antilipemic agent'/exp OR 'hydroxymethylglutaryl coenzyme A reductase inhibitor'/exp OR statins:ab,ti OR statin:ab,ti OR 'simvastatin'/exp OR simvastatin:ab,ti OR 'mevinolin'/exp OR lovastatin:ab,ti OR 'atorvastatin'/exp OR atorvastatin:ab,ti OR 'pravastatin'/exp OR pravastatin:ab,ti OR 'fluindostatin'/exp OR fluvastatin:ab,ti OR 'pitavastatin'/exp OR pitavastatin:ab,ti OR 'ezetimibe'/exp OR Ezetimibe:ab,ti OR 'nicotinic acid'/exp OR niacin:ab,ti OR 'fenofibrate'/exp OR fenofibrate:ab,ti OR 'fibric acid derivative'/exp OR "fibric acid":ab,ti OR "fibric acids":ab,ti OR fibrates:ab,ti OR fibrate:ab,ti OR 'gemfibrozil'/exp OR gemfibrozil:ab,ti OR 'colestipol'/exp OR 'colestyramine'/exp OR Colestipol:ab,ti OR Cholestyramine:ab,ti OR 'colesevelam'/exp OR colesevelam:ab,ti
#6	'diet therapy'/exp OR 'exercise'/exp OR 'kinesiotherapy'/exp OR 'low calory diet'/exp OR exercise:ab,ti OR "physical activity":ab,ti OR diet:ab,ti OR diets:ab,ti OR 'weight reduction'/exp OR "weight management":ab,ti OR 'behavior therapy'/exp OR 'cognitive therapy'/exp OR 'health education' OR counsel*:ab,ti OR 'counseling'/exp OR 'disease management'/exp OR 'lifestyle modification'/exp OR "lifestyle modification":ab,ti OR 'patient compliance'/exp OR "cognitive behavioral therapy":ab,ti OR adher*:ab,ti OR "self-monitoring":ab,ti OR 'recurrent disease'/exp/dm_pc OR "relapse prevention":ab,ti OR "skills training":ab,ti OR "motivational interviewing":ab,ti OR educat*:ab,ti
#7	'social support'/exp OR family:ab,ti OR peer:ab,ti
#8	'drug substitution'/exp OR substitut*:ab,ti switch:ab,ti OR switched:ab,ti OR switching:ab,ti OR change:ab,ti OR changed:ab,ti OR changing:ab,ti OR replace:ab,ti OR replaced:ab,ti OR replacing:ab,ti OR replacement:ab,ti OR abandon*:ab,ti
#9	#5 OR #6 OR #7 OR #8
#10	'controlled clinical trial'/exp OR randomized:ab,ti OR randomised:ab,ti OR randomization:ab,ti OR randomisation:ab,ti OR placebo:ab,ti OR randomly:ab,ti OR trial:ab,ti OR groups:ab,ti NOT ('case report'/exp OR 'case study'/exp OR 'editorial'/exp OR 'letter'/exp OR 'note'/exp)
#11	#4 AND #9 AND #10
#12	#11 AND [embase]/lim NOT [medline]/lim, Limits: English, Human

Table A-8. Embase search strings for KQ 4

Set #	Terms
#1	'schizophrenia'/exp OR 'bipolar disorder'/exp OR 'affective psychosis'/exp OR 'depressive psychosis'/exp OR 'manic depressive psychosis'/exp OR schizophrenia:ab,ti OR 'bipolar disorder':ab,ti OR 'psychotic disorders':ab,ti OR schizoaffective:ab,ti OR mania:ti OR manic:ti OR 'bipolar affective disorder':ab,ti OR 'serious mental illness':ab,ti OR 'severe mental illness':ab,ti OR 'severe psychiatric illness':ab,ti
#2	'cardiovascular disease'/exp AND 'hypertension'/exp OR 'hyperlipidemia'/exp OR hypertension:ab,ti OR ((cardiovascular:ab,ti OR heart:ab,ti OR coronary:ab,ti) AND (disease:ab,ti OR diseases:ab,ti OR risk:ab,ti))
#3	'chlorpromazine'/exp OR chlorpromazine:ab,ti OR thorazine:ab,ti OR 'fluphenazine'/exp OR fluphenazine:ab,ti OR 'haloperidol'/exp OR haloperidol:ab,ti OR haldol:ab,ti OR 'iloperidone'/exp OR iloperidone:ab,ti OR fanapt:ab,ti OR 'loxapine'/exp OR loxapine:ab,ti OR loxitane:ab,ti OR 'molindone'/exp OR molindone:ab,ti OR moban:ab,ti OR 'chlorpromazine'/exp OR chlorpromazine:ab,ti OR thorazine:ab,ti OR 'perphenazine'/exp OR perphenazine:ab,ti OR 'pimozide'/exp OR pimozide:ab,ti OR orap:ab,ti OR 'thioridazine'/exp OR thioridazine:ab,ti OR 'tiotixene'/exp OR thiothixene:ab,ti OR navane:ab,ti OR 'trifluoperazine'/exp OR trifluoperazine:ab,ti OR stelazine:ab,ti OR 'clozapine'/exp OR clozapine:ab,ti OR clozaril:ab,ti OR 'risperidone'/exp OR risperidone:ab,ti OR risperidal:ab,ti OR 'olanzapine'/exp OR olanzapine:ab,ti OR zyprexa:ab,ti OR 'quetiapine'/exp OR quetiapine:ab,ti OR seroquel:ab,ti OR 'ziprasidone'/exp OR ziprasidone:ab,ti OR geodon:ab,ti OR 'aripiprazole'/exp OR aripiprazole:ab,ti OR abilify:ab,ti OR "9-hydroxy-risperidone":ab,ti OR paliperidone:ab,ti OR invega:ab,ti OR 'neuroleptic agent'/exp OR antipsychotic:ab,ti OR antipsychotics:ab,ti
#4	#1 AND (#2 OR #3)

Set #	Terms
#5	'cardiovascular agent'/exp OR 'antilipemic agent'/exp OR 'nicotinic agent'/exp OR 'heparin'/exp OR 'warfarin'/exp OR 'low molecular weight heparin'/exp OR 'amfebutamone'/exp OR 'atorvastatin'/exp OR 'simvastatin'/exp OR 'pitavastatin'/exp OR 'rosuvastatin'/exp OR 'pravastatin'/exp OR 'colestyramine'/exp OR 'colesevelam'/exp OR 'colestipol'/exp OR 'ezetimibe'/exp OR 'fenofibrate'/exp OR 'fluindostatin'/exp OR 'mevinolin'/exp OR 'acebutolol'/exp OR 'aliskiren'/exp OR 'amiloride'/exp OR 'amlodipine'/exp OR 'atenolol'/exp OR 'azilsartan'/exp OR 'benazepril'/exp OR 'betaxolol'/exp OR 'bisoprolol'/exp OR 'candesartan'/exp OR 'carvedilol'/exp OR 'chlorothiazide'/exp OR 'chlortalidone'/exp OR 'clonidine'/exp OR 'diltiazem'/exp OR 'irbesartan'/exp OR 'isradipine'/exp OR 'labetalol'/exp OR 'lisinopril'/exp OR 'losartan'/exp OR 'metolazone'/exp OR 'metoprolol'/exp OR 'moexipril'/exp OR 'nebivolol'/exp OR 'nicardipine'/exp OR 'nifedipine'/exp OR 'nisoldipine'/exp OR 'olmesartan'/exp OR 'penbutolol'/exp OR 'perindopril'/exp OR 'pindolol'/exp OR 'prazosin'/exp OR 'propranolol'/exp OR 'quinapril'/exp OR 'ramipril'/exp OR 'telmisartan'/exp OR 'torasemide'/exp OR 'trandolapril'/exp OR 'valsartan'/exp OR 'verapamil'/exp OR Lipitor:ab,ti OR atorvastatin:ab,ti OR Caduet:ab,ti OR Prevalite:ab,ti OR cholestyramine:ab,ti OR Questran:ab,ti OR WelChol:ab,ti OR colesevelam:ab,ti OR Colestid:ab,ti OR colestipol:ab,ti OR Zetia:ab,ti OR ezetimibe:ab,ti OR Tricor:ab,ti OR fenofibrate:ab,ti OR Lescol:ab,ti OR fluvastatin:ab,ti OR Mevacor:ab,ti OR lovastatin:ab,ti OR Livalo:ab,ti OR pitavastatin:ab,ti OR Pravachol:ab,ti OR pravastatin:ab,ti OR Crestor:ab,ti OR rosuvastatin:ab,ti OR Zocor:ab,ti OR simvastatin:ab,ti OR Sectral:ab,ti OR Acebutolol:ab,ti OR Tekturna:ab,ti OR Aliskiren:ab,ti OR Tekamlo:ab,ti OR Valturna:ab,ti OR Midimor:ab,ti OR Amiloride:ab,ti OR Norvasc:ab,ti OR Amlodipine:ab,ti OR Caduet:ab,ti OR Lotrel:ab,ti OR Tenormin:ab,ti OR Atenolol:ab,ti OR Tenoretic:ab,ti OR Edarbi:ab,ti OR Azilsartan:ab,ti OR Lotensin:ab,ti OR Benazepril:ab,ti OR Kerlone:ab,ti OR Betaxolol:ab,ti OR Zebeta:ab,ti OR Bisoprolol:ab,ti OR Atacand:ab,ti OR Candesartan:ab,ti OR Coreg:ab,ti OR Carvedilol:ab,ti OR Diuril:ab,ti OR Chlorothiazide:ab,ti OR Thalitone:ab,ti OR Chlorthalidone:ab,ti OR Clorpres:ab,ti OR Catapres:ab,ti OR Clonidine:ab,ti OR Cardizem:ab,ti OR diltiazem:ab,ti OR Cartia:ab,ti OR Dilacor:ab,ti OR Dilt:ab,ti OR Diltia:ab,ti OR Matzim:ab,ti OR Taztia:ab,ti OR Tiamate:ab,ti OR Tiazac:ab,ti OR Avapro:ab,ti OR irbesartan:ab,ti OR Dynacirc:ab,ti OR isradipine:ab,ti OR Trandate:ab,ti OR labetalol:ab,ti OR Prinivil:ab,ti OR lisinopril:ab,ti OR Zestril:ab,ti OR Cozaar:ab,ti OR losartan:ab,ti OR Zaroxloyn:ab,ti OR metolazone:ab,ti OR Lopressor:ab,ti OR metoprolol:ab,ti OR Toprol:ab,ti OR Univasc:ab,ti OR moexipril:ab,ti OR Corgard:ab,ti OR nadalol:ab,ti OR Bystolic:ab,ti OR nebivolol:ab,ti OR Cardene:ab,ti OR nicardipine:ab,ti OR Procardia:ab,ti OR nifedipine:ab,ti OR Sular:ab,ti OR nisoldipine:ab,ti OR Benicar:ab,ti OR olmesartan:ab,ti OR Levitol:ab,ti OR penbutolol:ab,ti OR Aceon:ab,ti OR perindopril:ab,ti OR Pindolol:ab,ti OR pindolol:ab,ti OR Minipress:ab,ti OR prazosin:ab,ti OR Inderal:ab,ti OR propranolol:ab,ti OR Accupril:ab,ti OR quinapril:ab,ti OR Altace:ab,ti OR ramipril:ab,ti OR Micardis:ab,ti OR telmisartan:ab,ti OR Demadex:ab,ti OR torsemide:ab,ti OR Mavik:ab,ti OR trandolapril:ab,ti OR Diovan:ab,ti OR valsartan:ab,ti OR Calan:ab,ti OR verapamil:ab,ti OR Covera:ab,ti OR Isoptin:ab,ti OR Verelan:ab,ti OR heparin:ab,ti OR warfarin:ab,ti OR bupropion:ab,ti
#6	'smoking cessation'/exp OR 'smoking cessation program'/exp OR smoking:ab,ti OR tobacco:ab,ti OR 'diet therapy'/exp OR 'exercise'/exp OR 'kinesiotherapy'/exp OR 'low calory diet'/exp OR exercise:ab,ti OR "physical activity":ab,ti OR diet:ab,ti OR diets:ab,ti OR 'weight reduction'/exp OR "weight management":ab,ti OR 'behavior therapy'/exp OR 'cognitive therapy'/exp OR 'health education' OR counsel*:ab,ti OR 'counseling'/exp OR 'disease management'/exp OR 'lifestyle modification'/exp OR "lifestyle modification":ab,ti OR 'patient compliance'/exp OR "cognitive behavioral therapy":ab,ti OR adher*:ab,ti OR "self-monitoring":ab,ti OR 'recurrent disease'/exp/dm_pc OR "relapse prevention":ab,ti OR "skills training":ab,ti OR "motivational interviewing":ab,ti OR educat*:ab,ti
#7	'social support'/exp OR family:ab,ti OR peer:ab,ti
#8	'drug substitution'/exp OR substitut*:ab,ti switch:ab,ti OR switched:ab,ti OR switching:ab,ti OR change:ab,ti OR changed:ab,ti OR changing:ab,ti OR replace:ab,ti OR replaced:ab,ti OR replacing:ab,ti OR replacement:ab,ti OR abandon*:ab,ti
#9	#5 OR #6 OR #7 OR #8
#10	'controlled clinical trial'/exp OR randomized:ab,ti OR randomised:ab,ti OR randomization:ab,ti OR randomisation:ab,ti OR placebo:ab,ti OR randomly:ab,ti OR trial:ab,ti OR groups:ab,ti NOT ('case report'/exp OR 'case study'/exp OR 'editorial'/exp OR 'letter'/exp OR 'note'/exp)
#11	#4 AND #9 AND #10
#12	#11 AND [embase]/lim NOT [medline]/lim, Limits: English, Human

Cochrane Search Strategy (July 20, 2012)

Platform: Wiley

Database searched: Cochrane Database of Systematic Reviews (CDSR)

Table A-9. CDSR search strings for KQ 1

Set #	Terms
#1	MeSH descriptor Affective Disorders, Psychotic explode all trees OR MeSH descriptor Schizophrenia and Disorders with Psychotic Features explode all trees OR Schizophrenia:ti,ab OR schizoaffective:ti,ab OR mania:ti OR manic:ti OR "bipolar affective disorder":ti,ab OR "serious mental illness":ti,ab OR "severe mental illness":ti,ab OR "severe psychiatric illness":ti,ab OR ("depressive disorder":kw AND psychotic:ti,ab)
#2	MeSH descriptor Body Weights and Measures explode all trees OR overweight:ti,ab OR obesity:ti,ab OR obese:ti,ab OR weight:ti,ab OR "body mass index":ti,ab,kw OR bmi:ti,ab,kw
#3	MeSH descriptor Antipsychotic Agents explode all trees OR chlorpromazine:ti,ab,kw OR thorazine:ti,ab,kw OR fluphenazine:ti,ab,kw OR haloperidol:ti,ab,kw OR haldol:ti,ab,kw OR iloperidone:ti,ab,kw OR fanapt:ti,ab,kw OR loxapine:ti,ab,kw OR loxitane:ti,ab,kw OR molindone:ti,ab,kw OR moban:ti,ab,kw OR OR chlorpromazine:ti,ab,kw OR thorazine:ti,ab,kw OR perphenazine:ti,ab,kw OR pimozide:ti,ab,kw OR orap:ti,ab,kw OR thioridazine:ti,ab,kw OR thiothixene:ti,ab,kw OR navane:ti,ab,kw OR trifluoperazine:ti,ab,kw OR stelazine:ti,ab,kw OR clozapine:ti,ab,kw OR clozaril:ti,ab,kw OR risperidone:ti,ab,kw OR risperidal:ti,ab,kw OR olanzapine:ti,ab,kw OR zyprexa:ti,ab,kw OR quetiapine:ti,ab,kw OR seroquel:ti,ab,kw OR ziprasidone:ti,ab,kw OR geodon:ti,ab,kw OR OR aripiprazole:ti,ab,kw OR abilify:ti,ab,kw OR "9-hydroxy-risperidone":ti,ab,kw OR paliperidone:ti,ab,kw OR invega:ti,ab,kw OR antipsychotic:ti,ab,kw OR antipsychotics:ti,ab,kw
#4	#1 AND (#2 OR #3)
#5	MeSH descriptor Appetite Depressants explode all trees OR MeSH descriptor Anti-Obesity Agents explode all trees OR orlistat:ti,ab,kw OR OR topiramate:ti,ab,kw OR metformin:ti,ab,kw OR OR amantadine:ti,ab,kw
#6	MeSH descriptor Nutrition Therapy explode all trees OR 7 MeSH descriptor Exercise explode all trees OR MeSH descriptor Exercise Therapy explode all trees OR MeSH descriptor Exercise Movement Techniques explode all trees OR MeSH descriptor Recurrence explode all trees with qualifier: PC OR MeSH descriptor Behavior Therapy explode all trees OR MeSH descriptor Disease Management explode all trees OR MeSH descriptor Patient Compliance explode all trees OR MeSH descriptor Life Style explode all trees OR MeSH descriptor Counseling explode all trees OR exercise:ti,ab OR "physical activity":ti,ab OR diet:ti,ab OR diets:ti,ab OR "weight management":ti,ab OR health education[mesh] OR health promotion[mesh] OR counsel*:ti,ab OR "cognitive behavioral therapy":ti,ab OR "lifestyle modification":ti,ab OR adher*:ti,ab OR "self-monitoring":ti,ab OR "relapse prevention":ti,ab OR "skills training":ti,ab OR "motivational interviewing":ti,ab OR educat*:ti,ab
#7	MeSH descriptor Social Support explode all trees OR family:ti,ab OR peer:ti,ab
#8	MeSH descriptor Drug Substitution explode all trees OR substitut*:ti,ab OR switch:ti,ab OR switched:ti,ab OR switching:ti,ab OR change:ti,ab OR changed:ti,ab OR changing:ti,ab OR replace:ti,ab OR replaced:ti,ab OR replacing:ti,ab OR replacement:ti,ab OR abandon*:ti,ab
#9	#5 OR #6 OR #7 OR #8,
#10	#4 AND #9

Table A-10. CDSR search strings for KQ 2

Set #	Terms
#1	MeSH descriptor Affective Disorders, Psychotic explode all trees OR MeSH descriptor Schizophrenia and Disorders with Psychotic Features explode all trees OR Schizophrenia:ti,ab OR schizoaffective:ti,ab OR mania:ti OR manic:ti OR "bipolar affective disorder":ti,ab OR "serious mental illness":ti,ab OR "severe mental illness":ti,ab OR "severe psychiatric illness":ti,ab OR ("depressive disorder":kw AND psychotic:ti,ab)
#2	Diabetes mellitus[mesh] OR diabetes:ti,ab
#3	MeSH descriptor Antipsychotic Agents explode all trees OR chlorpromazine:ti,ab,kw OR thorazine:ti,ab,kw OR fluphenazine:ti,ab,kw OR haloperidol:ti,ab,kw OR haldol:ti,ab,kw OR iloperidone:ti,ab,kw OR fanapt:ti,ab,kw OR loxapine:ti,ab,kw OR loxitane:ti,ab,kw OR molindone:ti,ab,kw OR moban:ti,ab,kw OR OR chlorpromazine:ti,ab,kw OR thorazine:ti,ab,kw OR perphenazine:ti,ab,kw OR pimozide:ti,ab,kw OR orap:ti,ab,kw OR thioridazine:ti,ab,kw OR thiothixene:ti,ab,kw OR navane:ti,ab,kw OR trifluoperazine:ti,ab,kw OR stelazine:ti,ab,kw OR clozapine:ti,ab,kw OR clozaril:ti,ab,kw OR risperidone:ti,ab,kw OR risperidal:ti,ab,kw OR olanzapine:ti,ab,kw OR zyprexa:ti,ab,kw OR quetiapine:ti,ab,kw OR seroquel:ti,ab,kw OR ziprasidone:ti,ab,kw OR geodon:ti,ab,kw OR OR aripiprazole:ti,ab,kw OR abilify:ti,ab,kw OR "9-hydroxy-risperidone":ti,ab,kw OR paliperidone:ti,ab,kw OR invega:ti,ab,kw OR antipsychotic:ti,ab,kw OR antipsychotics:ti,ab,kw
#4	#1 AND (#2 OR #3)
#5	MeSH descriptor Hypoglycemic Agents explode all trees OR Byetta:ti,ab,kw OR exenatide:ti,ab,kw OR Symlin:ti,ab,kw OR pramlintide:ti,ab,kw OR Januvia:ti,ab,kw OR sitagliptin:ti,ab,kw OR Lantus:ti,ab,kw OR "insulin glargine":ti,ab,kw OR Onglyza:ti,ab,kw OR saxagliptin:ti,ab,kw OR Glyset:ti,ab,kw OR miglitol:ti,ab,kw OR Avandia:ti,ab,kw OR rosiglitazone:ti,ab,kw OR Actos:ti,ab,kw OR pioglitazone:ti,ab,kw OR Prandin:ti,ab,kw OR repaglinide:ti,ab,kw OR Starlix:ti,ab,kw OR nateglinide:ti,ab,kw OR Diabeta:ti,ab,kw OR glyburide:ti,ab,kw OR Amaryl:ti,ab,kw OR glimepiride:ti,ab,kw OR Glumetza:ti,ab,kw OR metformin:ti,ab,kw OR Riomet:ti,ab,kw OR Fortamet:ti,ab,kw OR Tradjenta:ti,ab,kw OR linagliptin:ti,ab,kw OR Victoza:ti,ab,kw OR liraglutide:ti,ab,kw OR WelChol:ti,ab,kw OR colesevelam:ti,ab,kw OR Cycloset:ti,ab,kw OR bromocriptine:ti,ab,kw OR Parlodel:ti,ab,kw
#6	MeSH descriptor Diabetes Mellitus explode all trees with qualifier: PC OR MeSH descriptor Recurrence explode all trees with qualifier: PC OR MeSH descriptor Behavior Therapy explode all trees OR MeSH descriptor Disease Management explode all trees OR MeSH descriptor Patient Compliance explode all trees OR MeSH descriptor Life Style explode all trees OR MeSH descriptor Counseling explode all trees OR "diabetes management":ti,ab OR counsel*:ti,ab OR "cognitive behavioral therapy":ti,ab OR "lifestyle modification":ti,ab OR adher*:ti,ab OR "self-monitoring":ti,ab OR "relapse prevention":ti,ab OR "skills training":ti,ab OR "motivational interviewing":ti,ab OR educat*:ti,ab
#7	MeSH descriptor Social Support explode all trees OR family:ti,ab OR peer:ti,ab
#8	MeSH descriptor Drug Substitution explode all trees OR substitut*:ti,ab OR switch:ti,ab OR switched:ti,ab OR switching:ti,ab OR change:ti,ab OR changed:ti,ab OR changing:ti,ab OR replace:ti,ab OR replaced:ti,ab OR replacing:ti,ab OR replacement:ti,ab OR abandon*:ti,ab
#9	#5 OR #6 OR #7 OR #8
#10	#4 AND #9

Table A-11. CDSR search strings for KQ 3

Set #	Terms
#1	MeSH descriptor Affective Disorders, Psychotic explode all trees OR MeSH descriptor Schizophrenia and Disorders with Psychotic Features explode all trees OR Schizophrenia:ti,ab OR schizoaffective:ti,ab OR mania:ti OR manic:ti OR "bipolar affective disorder":ti,ab OR "serious mental illness":ti,ab OR "severe mental illness":ti,ab OR "severe psychiatric illness":ti,ab OR ("depressive disorder":kw AND psychotic:ti,ab)
#2	MeSH descriptor Dyslipidemias explode all trees OR MeSH descriptor Hyperlipidemias explode all trees OR dyslipidemia:ti,ab OR dyslipidemias:ti,ab OR hyperlipidemia:ti,ab OR hyperlipidemias:ti,ab
#3	MeSH descriptor Antipsychotic Agents explode all trees OR chlorpromazine:ti,ab,kw OR thorazine:ti,ab,kw OR fluphenazine:ti,ab,kw OR haloperidol:ti,ab,kw OR haldol:ti,ab,kw OR iloperidone:ti,ab,kw OR fanapt:ti,ab,kw OR loxapine:ti,ab,kw OR loxitane:ti,ab,kw OR molindone:ti,ab,kw OR moban:ti,ab,kw OR OR chlorpromazine:ti,ab,kw OR thorazine:ti,ab,kw OR perphenazine:ti,ab,kw OR pimozide:ti,ab,kw OR orap:ti,ab,kw OR thioridazine:ti,ab,kw OR thiothixene:ti,ab,kw OR navane:ti,ab,kw OR trifluoperazine:ti,ab,kw OR stelazine:ti,ab,kw OR clozapine:ti,ab,kw OR clozaril:ti,ab,kw OR risperidone:ti,ab,kw OR risperidal:ti,ab,kw OR olanzapine:ti,ab,kw OR zyprexa:ti,ab,kw OR quetiapine:ti,ab,kw OR seroquel:ti,ab,kw OR ziprasidone:ti,ab,kw OR geodon:ti,ab,kw OR OR aripiprazole:ti,ab,kw OR abilify:ti,ab,kw OR "9-hydroxy-risperidone":ti,ab,kw OR paliperidone:ti,ab,kw OR invega:ti,ab,kw OR antipsychotic:ti,ab,kw OR antipsychotics:ti,ab,kw
#4	#1 AND (#2 OR #3)
#5	MeSH descriptor Hypolipidemic Agents explode all trees OR MeSH descriptor Hydroxymethylglutaryl-CoA Reductase Inhibitors explode all trees OR MeSH descriptor Fibric Acids explode all trees OR statins:ti,ab,kw OR statin:ti,ab,kw OR simvastatin:ti,ab,kw OR lovastatin:ti,ab,kw OR atorvastatin:ti,ab,kw OR pravastatin:ti,ab,kw OR fluvastatin:ti,ab,kw OR pitavastatin:ti,ab,kw OR Ezetimibe:ti,ab,kw OR niacin:ti,ab,kw OR fenofibrate:ti,ab,kw OR "fibric acid":ti,ab,kw OR "fibric acids":ti,ab,kw OR fibrates:ti,ab,kw OR fibrate:ti,ab,kw OR gemfibrozil:ti,ab,kw] OR Colestipol:ti,ab,kw OR Cholestyramine:ti,ab,kw OR colesevelam:ti,ab,kw
#6	MeSH descriptor Nutrition Therapy explode all trees OR 7 MeSH descriptor Exercise explode all trees OR MeSH descriptor Exercise Therapy explode all trees OR MeSH descriptor Exercise Movement Techniques explode all trees OR MeSH descriptor Recurrence explode all trees with qualifier: PC OR MeSH descriptor Behavior Therapy explode all trees OR MeSH descriptor Disease Management explode all trees OR MeSH descriptor Patient Compliance explode all trees OR MeSH descriptor Life Style explode all trees OR MeSH descriptor Counseling explode all trees OR exercise:ti,ab OR "physical activity":ti,ab OR diet:ti,ab OR diets:ti,ab OR "weight management":ti,ab OR health education[mesh] OR health promotion[mesh] OR counsel*:ti,ab OR "cognitive behavioral therapy":ti,ab OR "lifestyle modification":ti,ab OR adher*:ti,ab OR "self-monitoring":ti,ab OR "relapse prevention":ti,ab OR "skills training":ti,ab OR "motivational interviewing":ti,ab OR educat*:ti,ab
#7	MeSH descriptor Social Support explode all trees OR family:ti,ab OR peer:ti,ab
#8	MeSH descriptor Drug Substitution explode all trees OR substitut*:ti,ab OR switch:ti,ab OR switched:ti,ab OR switching:ti,ab OR change:ti,ab OR changed:ti,ab OR changing:ti,ab OR replace:ti,ab OR replaced:ti,ab OR replacing:ti,ab OR replacement:ti,ab OR abandon*:ti,ab
#9	#5 OR #6 OR #7 OR #8
#10	#4 AND #9

Table A-12. CDSR search strings for KQ 4

Set #	Terms
#1	MeSH descriptor Affective Disorders, Psychotic explode all trees OR MeSH descriptor Schizophrenia and Disorders with Psychotic Features explode all trees OR Schizophrenia:ti,ab OR schizoaffective:ti,ab OR mania:ti OR manic:ti OR "bipolar affective disorder":ti,ab OR "serious mental illness":ti,ab OR "severe mental illness":ti,ab OR "severe psychiatric illness":ti,ab OR ("depressive disorder":kw AND psychotic:ti,ab)
#2	MeSH descriptor Cardiovascular Diseases explode all trees OR MeSH descriptor Hyperlipidemias explode all trees OR hypertension:ti,ab OR ((cardiovascular:ti,ab OR heart:ti,ab OR coronary:ti,ab) AND (disease:ti,ab OR diseases:ti,ab OR risk:ti,ab))
#3	MeSH descriptor Antipsychotic Agents explode all trees OR chlorpromazine:ti,ab,kw OR thorazine:ti,ab,kw OR fluphenazine:ti,ab,kw OR haloperidol:ti,ab,kw OR haldol:ti,ab,kw OR iloperidone:ti,ab,kw OR fanapt:ti,ab,kw OR loxapine:ti,ab,kw OR loxitane:ti,ab,kw OR molindone:ti,ab,kw OR moban:ti,ab,kw OR OR chlorpromazine:ti,ab,kw OR thorazine:ti,ab,kw OR perphenazine:ti,ab,kw OR pimozide:ti,ab,kw OR orap:ti,ab,kw OR thioridazine:ti,ab,kw OR thiothixene:ti,ab,kw OR navane:ti,ab,kw OR trifluoperazine:ti,ab,kw OR stelazine:ti,ab,kw OR clozapine:ti,ab,kw OR clozaril:ti,ab,kw OR risperidone:ti,ab,kw OR risperidal:ti,ab,kw OR olanzapine:ti,ab,kw OR zyprexa:ti,ab,kw OR quetiapine:ti,ab,kw OR seroquel:ti,ab,kw OR ziprasidone:ti,ab,kw OR geodon:ti,ab,kw OR OR aripiprazole:ti,ab,kw OR abilify:ti,ab,kw OR "9-hydroxy-risperidone":ti,ab,kw OR paliperidone:ti,ab,kw OR invega:ti,ab,kw OR antipsychotic:ti,ab,kw OR antipsychotics:ti,ab,kw
#4	#1 AND (#2 OR #3)
#5	MeSH descriptor Antihypertensive Agents explode all trees OR MeSH descriptor Hypolipidemic Agents explode all trees OR MeSH descriptor Nicotinic Agonists explode all trees OR MeSH descriptor Cardiovascular Agents explode all trees OR Lipitor:ti,ab,kw OR atorvastatin:ti,ab,kw OR Caduet:ti,ab,kw OR Prevalite:ti,ab,kw OR cholestyramine:ti,ab,kw OR Questran:ti,ab,kw OR WelChol:ti,ab,kw OR colesevelam:ti,ab,kw OR Colestid:ti,ab,kw OR colestipol:ti,ab,kw OR Zetia:ti,ab,kw OR ezetimibe:ti,ab,kw OR Tricor:ti,ab,kw OR fenofibrate:ti,ab,kw OR Lescol:ti,ab,kw OR fluvastatin:ti,ab,kw OR Mevacor:ti,ab,kw OR lovastatin:ti,ab,kw OR Livalo:ti,ab,kw OR pitavastatin:ti,ab,kw OR Pravachol:ti,ab,kw OR pravastatin:ti,ab,kw OR Crestor:ti,ab,kw OR rosuvastatin:ti,ab,kw OR Zocor:ti,ab,kw OR simvastatin:ti,ab,kw OR Sectral:ti,ab,kw OR Acebutolol:ti,ab,kw OR Tekturna:ti,ab,kw OR Aliskiren:ti,ab,kw OR Tekamlo:ti,ab,kw OR Valturna:ti,ab,kw OR Midimor:ti,ab,kw OR Amiloride:ti,ab,kw OR Norvasc:ti,ab,kw OR Amlodipine:ti,ab,kw OR Caduet:ti,ab,kw OR Lotrel:ti,ab,kw OR Tenormin:ti,ab,kw OR Atenolol:ti,ab,kw OR Tenoretic:ti,ab,kw OR Edarbi:ti,ab,kw OR Azilsartan:ti,ab,kw OR Lotensin:ti,ab,kw OR Benazepril:ti,ab,kw OR Kerlone:ti,ab,kw OR Betaxolol:ti,ab,kw OR Zebeta:ti,ab,kw OR Bisoprolol:ti,ab,kw OR Atacand:ti,ab,kw OR Candesartan:ti,ab,kw OR Coreg:ti,ab,kw OR Carvedilol:ti,ab,kw OR Diuril:ti,ab,kw OR Chlorothiazide:ti,ab,kw OR Thalitone:ti,ab,kw OR Chlorthalidone:ti,ab,kw OR Clorpres:ti,ab,kw OR Catapres:ti,ab,kw OR Clonidine:ti,ab,kw OR Cardizem:ti,ab,kw OR diltiazem:ti,ab,kw OR Cartia:ti,ab,kw OR Dilacor:ti,ab,kw OR Dilt:ti,ab,kw OR Diltia:ti,ab,kw OR Matzim:ti,ab,kw OR Taztia:ti,ab,kw OR Tiamate:ti,ab,kw OR Tiazac:ti,ab,kw OR Avapro:ti,ab,kw OR irbesartan:ti,ab,kw OR Dynacirc:ti,ab,kw OR isradipine:ti,ab,kw OR Trandate:ti,ab,kw OR labetalol:ti,ab,kw OR Prinivil:ti,ab,kw OR lisinopril:ti,ab,kw OR Zestril:ti,ab,kw OR Cozaar:ti,ab,kw OR losartan:ti,ab,kw OR Zaroxloyn:ti,ab,kw OR metolazone:ti,ab,kw OR Lopressor:ti,ab,kw OR metoprolol:ti,ab,kw OR Toprol:ti,ab,kw OR Univasc:ti,ab,kw OR moexipril:ti,ab,kw OR Corgard:ti,ab,kw OR nadalol:ti,ab,kw OR Bystolic:ti,ab,kw OR nebivolol:ti,ab,kw OR Cardene:ti,ab,kw OR nicardipine:ti,ab,kw OR Procardia:ti,ab,kw OR nifedipine:ti,ab,kw OR Sular:ti,ab,kw OR nisoldipine:ti,ab,kw OR Benicar:ti,ab,kw OR olmesartan:ti,ab,kw OR Levitol:ti,ab,kw OR penbutolol:ti,ab,kw OR Aceon:ti,ab,kw OR perindopril:ti,ab,kw OR Pindolol:ti,ab,kw OR pindolol:ti,ab,kw OR Minipress:ti,ab,kw OR prazosin:ti,ab,kw OR Inderal:ti,ab,kw OR propranolol:ti,ab,kw OR Accupril:ti,ab,kw OR quinapril:ti,ab,kw OR Altace:ti,ab,kw OR ramipril:ti,ab,kw OR Micardis:ti,ab,kw OR telmisartan:ti,ab,kw OR Demadex:ti,ab,kw OR torsemide:ti,ab,kw OR Mavik:ti,ab,kw OR trandolapril:ti,ab,kw OR Diovan:ti,ab,kw OR valsartan:ti,ab,kw OR Calan:ti,ab,kw OR verapamil:ti,ab,kw OR Covera:ti,ab,kw OR Isoptin:ti,ab,kw OR Verelan:ti,ab,kw OR heparin:ti,ab,kw OR warfarin:ti,ab,kw OR bupropion:ti,ab,kw

Set #	Terms
#6	MeSH descriptor Smoking Cessation explode all trees MeSH descriptor Nutrition Therapy explode all trees OR 7 MeSH descriptor Exercise explode all trees OR MeSH descriptor Exercise Therapy explode all trees OR MeSH descriptor Exercise Movement Techniques explode all trees OR MeSH descriptor Recurrence explode all trees with qualifier: PC OR MeSH descriptor Behavior Therapy explode all trees OR MeSH descriptor Disease Management explode all trees OR MeSH descriptor Patient Compliance explode all trees OR MeSH descriptor Life Style explode all trees OR MeSH descriptor Counseling explode all trees OR exercise:ti,ab OR "physical activity":ti,ab OR diet:ti,ab OR diets:ti,ab OR "weight management":ti,ab OR health education[mesh] OR health promotion[mesh] OR counsel*:ti,ab OR "cognitive behavioral therapy":ti,ab OR "lifestyle modification":ti,ab OR adher*:ti,ab OR "self-monitoring":ti,ab OR "relapse prevention":ti,ab OR "skills training":ti,ab OR "motivational interviewing":ti,ab OR educat*:ti,ab OR smoking:ti,ab OR tobacco:ti,ab
#7	MeSH descriptor Social Support explode all trees OR family:ti,ab OR peer:ti,ab
#8	MeSH descriptor Drug Substitution explode all trees OR substitut*:ti,ab OR switch:ti,ab OR switched:ti,ab OR switching:ti,ab OR change:ti,ab OR changed:ti,ab OR changing:ti,ab OR replace:ti,ab OR replaced:ti,ab OR replacing:ti,ab OR replacement:ti,ab OR abandon*:ti,ab
#9	#5 OR #6 OR #7 OR #8
#11	#4 AND #9

PsycINFO® Search Strategy (July 20, 2012)

Table A-13. PsycINFO search strings for KQ 1

Set #	Terms
#1	((((DE "Schizophrenia" OR DE "Acute Schizophrenia" OR DE "Catatonic Schizophrenia" OR DE "Childhood Schizophrenia" OR DE "Paranoid Schizophrenia" OR DE "Process Schizophrenia" OR DE "Schizophrenia (Disorganized Type)" OR DE "Schizophreniform Disorder" OR DE "Undifferentiated Schizophrenia") OR (DE "Bipolar Disorder" OR DE "Cyclothymic Personality")) OR (DE "Schizoaffective Disorder")) OR (DE "Psychosis")) OR (DE "Major Depression" OR DE "Anaclitic Depression" OR DE "Dysthymic Disorder" OR DE "Endogenous Depression" OR DE "Postpartum Depression" OR DE "Reactive Depression" OR DE "Recurrent Depression" OR DE "Treatment Resistant Depression") AND ((TI psychotic OR AB psychotic)) OR TI (mania OR manic OR Schizophrenia OR "bipolar disorder" OR "psychotic disorders" OR schizoaffective OR "bipolar affective disorder" OR "serious mental illness" OR "severe mental illness" OR "severe psychiatric illness") OR AB (Schizophrenia OR "bipolar disorder" OR "psychotic disorders" OR schizoaffective OR "bipolar affective disorder" OR "serious mental illness" OR "severe mental illness" OR "severe psychiatric illness")
#2	DE "Body Weight" OR DE "Birth Weight" OR DE "Overweight" OR DE "Underweight" OR DE "Weight Gain" OR DE "Weight Loss" OR TI (overweight OR obesity OR obese OR weight OR "body mass index" OR bmi) OR AB (overweight OR obesity OR obese OR weight OR "body mass index" OR bmi)

Set #	Terms
#3	DE "Chlorpromazine" OR DE "Fluphenazine" OR DE "Haloperidol" OR DE "Loxapine" OR DE "Molindone" OR DE "Perphenazine" OR DE "Pimozide" OR DE "Thioridazine" OR DE "Thiothixene" OR DE "Trifluoperazine" OR DE "Clozapine" OR DE "Risperidone" OR DE "Olanzapine" OR DE "Quetiapine" OR DE "Aripiprazole" OR DE "Neuroleptic Drugs" OR DE "Aripiprazole" OR DE "Clozapine" OR DE "Molindone" OR DE "Nialamide" OR DE "Olanzapine" OR DE "Quetiapine" OR DE "Reserpine" OR DE "Risperidone" OR DE "Spiroperidol" OR DE "Sulpiride" OR DE "Tetrabenazine" OR TI (chlorpromazine OR thorazine OR fluphenazine OR haloperidol OR haldol OR iloperidone OR fanapt OR loxapine OR loxitane OR molindone OR moban OR chlorpromazine OR thorazine OR perphenazine OR pimozide OR orap OR thioridazine OR thiothixene OR navane OR trifluoperazine OR stelazine OR clozapine OR clozaril OR risperidone OR risperidal OR olanzapine OR zyprexa OR quetiapine OR seroquel OR ziprasidone OR geodon OR aripiprazole OR abilify OR "9-hydroxy-risperidone" OR paliperidone OR invega OR antipsychotic OR antipsychotics) OR AB (chlorpromazine OR thorazine OR fluphenazine OR haloperidol OR haldol OR iloperidone OR fanapt OR loxapine OR loxitane OR molindone OR moban OR chlorpromazine OR thorazine OR perphenazine OR pimozide OR orap OR thioridazine OR thiothixene OR navane OR trifluoperazine OR stelazine OR clozapine OR clozaril OR risperidone OR risperidal OR olanzapine OR zyprexa OR quetiapine OR seroquel OR ziprasidone OR geodon OR aripiprazole OR abilify OR "9-hydroxy-risperidone" OR paliperidone OR invega OR antipsychotic OR antipsychotics)
#4	#1 AND (#2 OR #3)
#5	(DE "Amantadine") OR (DE "Appetite Depressing Drugs" OR DE "Amphetamine" OR DE "Dextroamphetamine" OR DE "Fenfluramine" OR DE "Phenmetrazine") OR TI (orlistat OR topiramate OR metformin OR amantadine OR (Appetite AND (drugs OR drug)) OR ((antiobesity OR anti-obesity) AND (drugs OR drug))) OR AB (orlistat OR topiramate OR metformin OR amantadine OR (Appetite AND (drugs OR drug)) OR ((antiobesity OR anti-obesity) AND (drugs OR drug)))
#6	DE "Diets" OR DE "Aerobic Exercise" OR DE "Weightlifting" OR DE "Yoga" OR DE "Movement Therapy" OR DE "Physical Activity" OR DE "Exercise" OR DE "Behavior Therapy" OR DE "Aversion Therapy" OR DE "Conversion Therapy" OR DE "Dialectical Behavior Therapy" OR DE "Exposure Therapy" OR DE "Implosive Therapy" OR DE "Reciprocal Inhibition Therapy" OR DE "Response Cost" OR DE "Systematic Desensitization Therapy" OR DE "Cognitive Behavior Therapy" OR DE "Acceptance and Commitment Therapy" OR DE "Health Education" OR DE "Drug Education" OR DE "Sex Education" AND DE "Counseling" OR DE "Educational Counseling" OR DE "Group Counseling" OR DE "Microcounseling" OR DE "Peer Counseling" OR DE "Psychotherapeutic Counseling" OR DE "Family Therapy" OR DE "Disease Management" OR DE "Lifestyle Changes" OR DE "Treatment Compliance" OR DE "Relapse Prevention" OR DE "Motivational Interviewing" OR DE "Self Monitoring" OR DE "Weight Loss" OR TI (exercise OR "physical activity" OR diet OR diets OR "weight management" OR counsel* OR "cognitive behavioral therapy" OR "lifestyle modification" OR adher* OR "self-monitoring" OR "relapse prevention" OR "skills training" OR "motivational interviewing" OR educat*) OR AB (exercise OR "physical activity" OR diet OR diets OR "weight management" OR counsel* OR "cognitive behavioral therapy" OR "lifestyle modification" OR adher* OR "self-monitoring" OR "relapse prevention" OR "skills training" OR "motivational interviewing" OR educat*)
#7	DE "Social Support" OR TI (family OR peer) OR AB (family OR peer)
#8	TI (substitut* OR switch OR switched OR switching OR change OR changed OR changing OR replace OR replaced OR replacing OR replacement OR abandon*) AND AB (substitut* OR switch OR switched OR switching OR change OR changed OR changing OR replace OR replaced OR replacing OR replacement OR abandon*)
#9	#8 AND #3
#10	#5 OR #6 OR #7 OR #9
#11	#4 AND #10 Limiters - English; Methodology: TREATMENT OUTCOME/CLINICAL TRIAL

Table A-14. PsycINFO search strings for KQ 2

Set #	Terms
#1	(((DE "Schizophrenia" OR DE "Acute Schizophrenia" OR DE "Catatonic Schizophrenia" OR DE "Childhood Schizophrenia" OR DE "Paranoid Schizophrenia" OR DE "Process Schizophrenia" OR DE "Schizophrenia (Disorganized Type)" OR DE "Schizophreniform Disorder" OR DE "Undifferentiated Schizophrenia") OR (DE "Bipolar Disorder" OR DE "Cyclothymic Personality")) OR (DE "Schizoaffective Disorder")) OR (DE "Psychosis") OR (DE "Major Depression" OR DE "Anaclitic Depression" OR DE "Dysthymic Disorder" OR DE "Endogenous Depression" OR DE "Postpartum Depression" OR DE "Reactive Depression" OR DE "Recurrent Depression" OR DE "Treatment Resistant Depression") AND ((TI psychotic OR AB psychotic)) OR TI (mania OR manic OR Schizophrenia OR "bipolar disorder" OR "psychotic disorders" OR schizoaffective OR "bipolar affective disorder" OR "serious mental illness" OR "severe mental illness" OR "severe psychiatric illness") OR AB (Schizophrenia OR "bipolar disorder" OR "psychotic disorders" OR schizoaffective OR "bipolar affective disorder" OR "serious mental illness" OR "severe mental illness" OR "severe psychiatric illness")
#2	DE "Diabetes Mellitus" OR TI diabetes OR AB diabetes
#3	DE "Chlorpromazine" OR DE "Fluphenazine" OR DE "Haloperidol" OR DE "Loxapine" OR DE "Molindone" OR DE "Perphenazine" OR DE "Pimozide" OR DE "Thioridazine" OR DE "Thiothixene" OR DE "Trifluoperazine" OR DE "Clozapine" OR DE "Risperidone" OR DE "Olanzapine" OR DE "Quetiapine" OR DE "Aripiprazole" OR DE "Neuroleptic Drugs" OR DE "Aripiprazole" OR DE "Clozapine" OR DE "Molindone" OR DE "Nialamide" OR DE "Olanzapine" OR DE "Quetiapine" OR DE "Reserpine" OR DE "Risperidone" OR DE "Spiroperidol" OR DE "Sulpiride" OR DE "Tetrabenazine" OR TI (chlorpromazine OR thorazine OR fluphenazine OR haloperidol OR haldol OR iloperidone OR fanapt OR loxapine OR loxitane OR molindone OR moban OR chlorpromazine OR thorazine OR perphenazine OR pimozide OR orap OR thioridazine OR thiothixene OR navane OR trifluoperazine OR stelazine OR clozapine OR clozaril OR risperidone OR risperidal OR olanzapine OR zyprexa OR quetiapine OR seroquel OR ziprasidone OR geodon OR aripiprazole OR abilify OR "9-hydroxy-risperidone" OR paliperidone OR invega OR antipsychotic OR antipsychotics) OR AB (chlorpromazine OR thorazine OR fluphenazine OR haloperidol OR haldol OR iloperidone OR fanapt OR loxapine OR loxitane OR molindone OR moban OR chlorpromazine OR thorazine OR perphenazine OR pimozide OR orap OR thioridazine OR thiothixene OR navane OR trifluoperazine OR stelazine OR clozapine OR clozaril OR risperidone OR risperidal OR olanzapine OR zyprexa OR quetiapine OR seroquel OR ziprasidone OR geodon OR aripiprazole OR abilify OR "9-hydroxy-risperidone" OR paliperidone OR invega OR antipsychotic OR antipsychotics)
#4	#1 AND (#2 OR #3)
#5	TI (Byetta OR exenatide OR pramlintide OR Symlin OR Januvia OR sitagliptin OR glargine OR Lantus OR Onglyza OR saxagliptin OR miglitol OR Glyset OR Avandia OR rosiglitazone OR Actos OR pioglitazone OR Prandin OR repaglinide OR Starlix OR nateglinide OR glyburide OR Diabeta OR glyburide OR glimepiride OR Amaryl OR metformin OR Glumetza OR Riomet OR Fortamet OR Tradjenta OR linagliptin OR Victoza OR liraglutide OR colesevelam OR WelChol OR Cycloset OR bromocriptine OR Parlodel OR Hypoglycemic) OR AB (Byetta OR exenatide OR pramlintide OR Symlin OR Januvia OR sitagliptin OR glargine OR Lantus OR Onglyza OR saxagliptin OR miglitol OR Glyset OR Avandia OR rosiglitazone OR Actos OR pioglitazone OR Prandin OR repaglinide OR Starlix OR nateglinide OR glyburide OR Diabeta OR glyburide OR glimepiride OR Amaryl OR metformin OR Glumetza OR Riomet OR Fortamet OR Tradjenta OR linagliptin OR Victoza OR liraglutide OR colesevelam OR WelChol OR Cycloset OR bromocriptine OR Parlodel OR Hypoglycemic)

Set #	Terms
#6	TI diabetes management OR AB diabetes management OR DE "Behavior Therapy" OR DE "Aversion Therapy" OR DE "Conversion Therapy" OR DE "Dialectical Behavior Therapy" OR DE "Exposure Therapy" OR DE "Implosive Therapy" OR DE "Reciprocal Inhibition Therapy" OR DE "Response Cost" OR DE "Systematic Desensitization Therapy" OR DE "Cognitive Behavior Therapy" OR DE "Acceptance and Commitment Therapy" OR DE "Health Education" OR DE "Drug Education" OR DE "Sex Education" AND DE "Counseling" OR DE "Educational Counseling" OR DE "Group Counseling" OR DE "Microcounseling" OR DE "Peer Counseling" OR DE "Psychotherapeutic Counseling" OR DE "Family Therapy" OR DE "Disease Management" OR DE "Lifestyle Changes" OR DE "Treatment Compliance" OR DE "Relapse Prevention" OR DE "Motivational Interviewing" OR DE "Self Monitoring" OR DE "Weight Loss" OR TI (counsel* OR "cognitive behavioral therapy" OR "lifestyle modification" OR adher* OR "self-monitoring" OR "relapse prevention" OR "skills training" OR "motivational interviewing" OR educat*) OR AB (counsel* OR "cognitive behavioral therapy" OR "lifestyle modification" OR adher* OR "self-monitoring" OR "relapse prevention" OR "skills training" OR "motivational interviewing" OR educat*)
#7	DE "Social Support" OR TI (family OR peer) OR AB (family OR peer)
#8	TI (substitut* OR switch OR switched OR switching OR change OR changed OR changing OR replace OR replaced OR replacing OR replacement OR abandon*) AND AB (substitut* OR switch OR switched OR switching OR change OR changed OR changing OR replace OR replaced OR replacing OR replacement OR abandon*)
#9	#8 AND #3
#10	#5 OR #6 OR #7 OR #9
#11	#4 AND #10 Limiters - English; Methodology: TREATMENT OUTCOME/CLINICAL TRIAL

Table A-15. PsycINFO search strings for KQ 3

Set #	Terms
#1	((((DE "Schizophrenia" OR DE "Acute Schizophrenia" OR DE "Catatonic Schizophrenia" OR DE "Childhood Schizophrenia" OR DE "Paranoid Schizophrenia" OR DE "Process Schizophrenia" OR DE "Schizophrenia (Disorganized Type)" OR DE "Schizophreniform Disorder" OR DE "Undifferentiated Schizophrenia") OR (DE "Bipolar Disorder" OR DE "Cyclothymic Personality")) OR (DE "Schizoaffective Disorder")) OR (DE "Psychosis") OR (DE "Major Depression" OR DE "Anaclitic Depression" OR DE "Dysthymic Disorder" OR DE "Endogenous Depression" OR DE "Postpartum Depression" OR DE "Reactive Depression" OR DE "Recurrent Depression" OR DE "Treatment Resistant Depression") AND ((TI psychotic OR AB psychotic)) OR TI (mania OR manic OR Schizophrenia OR "bipolar disorder" OR "psychotic disorders" OR schizoaffective OR "bipolar affective disorder" OR "serious mental illness" OR "severe mental illness" OR "severe psychiatric illness") OR AB (Schizophrenia OR "bipolar disorder" OR "psychotic disorders" OR schizoaffective OR "bipolar affective disorder" OR "serious mental illness" OR "severe mental illness" OR "severe psychiatric illness")
#2	TI (Dyslipidemias OR Hyperlipidemias OR dyslipidemia OR hyperlipidemia) OR AB (Dyslipidemias OR Hyperlipidemias OR dyslipidemia OR hyperlipidemia)
#3	DE "Chlorpromazine" OR DE "Fluphenazine" OR DE "Haloperidol" OR DE "Loxapine" OR DE "Molindone" OR DE "Perphenazine" OR DE "Pimozide" OR DE "Thioridazine" OR DE "Thiothixene" OR DE "Trifluoperazine" OR DE "Clozapine" OR DE "Risperidone" OR DE "Olanzapine" OR DE "Quetiapine" OR DE "Aripiprazole" OR DE "Neuroleptic Drugs" OR DE "Aripiprazole" OR DE "Clozapine" OR DE "Molindone" OR DE "Nialamide" OR DE "Olanzapine" OR DE "Quetiapine" OR DE "Reserpine" OR DE "Risperidone" OR DE "Spiroperidol" OR DE "Sulpiride" OR DE "Tetrabenazine" OR TI (chlorpromazine OR thorazine OR fluphenazine OR haloperidol OR haldol OR iloperidone OR fanapt OR loxapine OR loxitane OR molindone OR moban OR chlorpromazine OR thorazine OR perphenazine OR pimozide OR orap OR thioridazine OR thiothixene OR navane OR trifluoperazine OR stelazine OR clozapine OR clozaril OR risperidone OR risperidal OR olanzapine OR zyprexa OR quetiapine OR seroquel OR ziprasidone OR geodon OR aripiprazole OR abilify OR "9-hydroxy-risperidone" OR paliperidone OR invega OR antipsychotic OR antipsychotics) OR AB (chlorpromazine OR thorazine OR fluphenazine OR haloperidol OR haldol OR iloperidone OR fanapt OR loxapine OR loxitane OR molindone OR moban OR chlorpromazine OR thorazine OR perphenazine OR pimozide OR orap OR thioridazine OR thiothixene OR navane OR trifluoperazine OR stelazine OR clozapine OR clozaril OR risperidone OR risperidal OR olanzapine OR zyprexa OR quetiapine OR seroquel OR ziprasidone OR geodon OR aripiprazole OR abilify OR "9-hydroxy-risperidone" OR paliperidone OR invega OR antipsychotic OR antipsychotics)

Set #	Terms
#4	#1 AND (#2 OR #3)
#5	TI (Hypolipidemic OR Hydroxymethylglutaryl-CoA Reductase Inhibitors OR statins OR statin OR simvastatin OR lovastatin OR atorvastatin OR pravastatin OR fluvastatin OR pitavastatin OR Ezetimibe OR niacin OR fenofibrate OR Fibric Acids OR fibric acid OR fibrates OR fibrate OR gemfibrozil OR Colestipol OR Cholestyramine Resin OR Cholestyramine OR colesevelam) OR AB (Hypolipidemic OR Hydroxymethylglutaryl-CoA Reductase Inhibitors OR statins OR statin OR simvastatin OR lovastatin OR atorvastatin OR pravastatin OR fluvastatin OR pitavastatin OR Ezetimibe OR niacin OR fenofibrate OR Fibric Acids OR fibric acid OR fibrates OR fibrate OR gemfibrozil OR Colestipol OR Cholestyramine Resin OR Cholestyramine OR colesevelam) OR KW (Hypolipidemic OR Hydroxymethylglutaryl-CoA Reductase Inhibitors OR statins OR statin OR simvastatin OR lovastatin OR atorvastatin OR pravastatin OR fluvastatin OR pitavastatin OR Ezetimibe OR niacin OR fenofibrate OR Fibric Acids OR fibric acid OR fibrates OR fibrate OR gemfibrozil OR Colestipol OR Cholestyramine Resin OR Cholestyramine OR colesevelam)
#6	DE "Diets" OR DE "Aerobic Exercise" OR DE "Weightlifting" OR DE "Yoga" OR DE "Movement Therapy" OR DE "Physical Activity" OR DE "Exercise" OR DE "Behavior Therapy" OR DE "Aversion Therapy" OR DE "Conversion Therapy" OR DE "Dialectical Behavior Therapy" OR DE "Exposure Therapy" OR DE "Implosive Therapy" OR DE "Reciprocal Inhibition Therapy" OR DE "Response Cost" OR DE "Systematic Desensitization Therapy" OR DE "Cognitive Behavior Therapy" OR DE "Acceptance and Commitment Therapy" OR DE "Health Education" OR DE "Drug Education" OR DE "Sex Education" AND DE "Counseling" OR DE "Educational Counseling" OR DE "Group Counseling" OR DE "Microcounseling" OR DE "Peer Counseling" OR DE "Psychotherapeutic Counseling" OR DE "Family Therapy" OR DE "Disease Management" OR DE "Lifestyle Changes" OR DE "Treatment Compliance" OR DE "Relapse Prevention" OR DE "Motivational Interviewing" OR DE "Self Monitoring" OR DE "Weight Loss" OR TI (exercise OR "physical activity" OR diet OR diets OR "weight management" OR counsel* OR "cognitive behavioral therapy" OR "lifestyle modification" OR adher* OR "self-monitoring" OR "relapse prevention" OR "skills training" OR "motivational interviewing" OR educat*) OR AB (exercise OR "physical activity" OR diet OR diets OR "weight management" OR counsel* OR "cognitive behavioral therapy" OR "lifestyle modification" OR adher* OR "self-monitoring" OR "relapse prevention" OR "skills training" OR "motivational interviewing" OR educat*)
#7	DE "Social Support" OR TI (family OR peer) OR AB (family OR peer)
#8	TI (substitut* OR switch OR switched OR switching OR change OR changed OR changing OR replace OR replaced OR replacing OR replacement OR abandon*) AND AB (substitut* OR switch OR switched OR switching OR change OR changed OR changing OR replace OR replaced OR replacing OR replacement OR abandon*)
#9	#8 AND #3
#10	#5 OR #6 OR #7 OR #9
#11	#4 AND #10 Limiters - English; Methodology: TREATMENT OUTCOME/CLINICAL TRIAL

Table A-16. PsycINFO search strings for KQ 4

Set #	Terms
#1	((((DE "Schizophrenia" OR DE "Acute Schizophrenia" OR DE "Catatonic Schizophrenia" OR DE "Childhood Schizophrenia" OR DE "Paranoid Schizophrenia" OR DE "Process Schizophrenia" OR DE "Schizophrenia (Disorganized Type)" OR DE "Schizophreniform Disorder" OR DE "Undifferentiated Schizophrenia") OR (DE "Bipolar Disorder" OR DE "Cyclothymic Personality")) OR (DE "Schizoaffective Disorder")) OR (DE "Psychosis")) OR (DE "Major Depression" OR DE "Anaclitic Depression" OR DE "Dysthymic Disorder" OR DE "Endogenous Depression" OR DE "Postpartum Depression" OR DE "Reactive Depression" OR DE "Recurrent Depression" OR DE "Treatment Resistant Depression") AND ((TI psychotic OR AB psychotic)) OR TI (mania OR manic OR Schizophrenia OR "bipolar disorder" OR "psychotic disorders" OR schizoaffective OR "bipolar affective disorder" OR "serious mental illness" OR "severe mental illness" OR "severe psychiatric illness") OR AB (Schizophrenia OR "bipolar disorder" OR "psychotic disorders" OR schizoaffective OR "bipolar affective disorder" OR "serious mental illness" OR "severe mental illness" OR "severe psychiatric illness")

Set #	Terms
#2	DE "Cardiovascular Disorders" OR DE "Aneurysms" OR DE "Arteriosclerosis" OR DE "Blood Pressure Disorders" OR DE "Cerebrovascular Disorders" OR DE "Embolisms" OR DE "Heart Disorders" OR DE "Hemorrhage" OR DE "Hypertension" OR DE "Ischemia" OR DE "Thromboses" OR TI (hypertension OR ((cardiovascular OR heart OR coronary) AND (disease OR diseases OR risk))) OR AB (hypertension OR ((cardiovascular OR heart OR coronary) AND (disease OR diseases OR risk)))
#3	DE "Chlorpromazine" OR DE "Fluphenazine" OR DE "Haloperidol" OR DE "Loxapine" OR DE "Molindone" OR DE "Perphenazine" OR DE "Pimozide" OR DE "Thioridazine" OR DE "Thiothixene" OR DE "Trifluoperazine" OR DE "Clozapine" OR DE "Risperidone" OR DE "Olanzapine" OR DE "Quetiapine" OR DE "Aripiprazole" OR DE "Neuroleptic Drugs" OR DE "Aripiprazole" OR DE "Clozapine" OR DE "Molindone" OR DE "Nialamide" OR DE "Olanzapine" OR DE "Quetiapine" OR DE "Reserpine" OR DE "Risperidone" OR DE "Spiroperidol" OR DE "Sulpiride" OR DE "Tetrabenazine" OR TI (chlorpromazine OR thorazine OR fluphenazine OR haloperidol OR haldol OR iloperidone OR fanapt OR loxapine OR loxitane OR molindone OR moban OR chlorpromazine OR thorazine OR perphenazine OR pimozide OR orap OR thioridazine OR thiothixene OR navane OR trifluoperazine OR stelazine OR clozapine OR clozaril OR risperidone OR risperidal OR olanzapine OR zyprexa OR quetiapine OR seroquel OR ziprasidone OR geodon OR aripiprazole OR abilify OR "9-hydroxy-risperidone" OR paliperidone OR invega OR antipsychotic OR antipsychotics) OR AB (chlorpromazine OR thorazine OR fluphenazine OR haloperidol OR haldol OR iloperidone OR fanapt OR loxapine OR loxitane OR molindone OR moban OR chlorpromazine OR thorazine OR perphenazine OR pimozide OR orap OR thioridazine OR thiothixene OR navane OR trifluoperazine OR stelazine OR clozapine OR clozaril OR risperidone OR risperidal OR olanzapine OR zyprexa OR quetiapine OR seroquel OR ziprasidone OR geodon OR aripiprazole OR abilify OR "9-hydroxy-risperidone" OR paliperidone OR invega OR antipsychotic OR antipsychotics)
#4	#1 AND (#2 OR #3)

Set #	Terms
#5	TI (Lipitor OR atorvastatin OR Caduet OR Prevalite OR cholestyramine OR Questran OR WelChol OR colesevelam OR Colestid OR colestipol OR Zetia OR ezetimibe OR Tricor OR fenofibrate OR Lescol OR fluvastatin OR Mevacor OR lovastatin OR Livalo OR pitavastatin OR Pravachol OR pravastatin OR Crestor OR rosuvastatin OR Zocor OR simvastatin OR Sectral OR Acebutolol OR Tekturna OR Aliskiren OR Tekamlo OR Valturna OR Midimor OR Amiloride OR Norvasc OR Amlodipine OR Caduet OR Lotrel OR Tenormin OR Atenolol OR Tenoretic OR Edarbi OR Azilsartan OR Lotensin OR Benazepril OR Kerlone OR Betaxolol OR Zebeta OR Bisoprolol OR Atacand OR Candesartan OR Coreg OR Carvedilol OR Diuril OR Chlorothiazide OR Thalitone OR Chlorthalidone OR Clorpres OR Catapres OR Clonidine OR Cardizem OR diltiazem OR Cartia OR Dilacor OR Dilt OR Diltia OR Matzim OR Taztia OR Tiamate OR Tiazac OR Avapro OR irbesartan OR Dynacirc OR isradipine OR Trandate OR labetalol OR Prinivil OR lisinopril OR Zestril OR Cozaar OR losartan OR Zaroxloyn OR metolazone OR Lopressor OR metoprolol OR Toprol OR Univasc OR moexipril OR Corgard OR nadalol OR Bystolic OR nebivolol OR Cardene OR nicardipine OR Procardia OR nifedipine OR Sular OR nisoldipine OR Benicar OR olmesartan OR Levitol OR penbutolol OR Aceon OR perindopril OR Pindolol OR pindolol OR Minipress OR prazosin OR Inderal OR propranolol OR Accupril OR quinapril OR Altace OR ramipril OR Micardis OR telmisartan OR Demadex OR torsemide OR Mavik OR trandolapril OR Diovan OR valsartan OR Calan OR verapamil OR Covera OR Isoptin OR Verelan OR Antihypertensive OR antihypertensives OR Hypolipidemic OR hypolipidemics OR "Nicotinic Agonists" OR Heparin OR Warfarin OR anticoagulant OR anticoagulants OR bupropion) OR AB (Lipitor OR atorvastatin OR Caduet OR Prevalite OR cholestyramine OR Questran OR WelChol OR colesevelam OR Colestid OR colestipol OR Zetia OR ezetimibe OR Tricor OR fenofibrate OR Lescol OR fluvastatin OR Mevacor OR lovastatin OR Livalo OR pitavastatin OR Pravachol OR pravastatin OR Crestor OR rosuvastatin OR Zocor OR simvastatin OR Sectral OR Acebutolol OR Tekturna OR Aliskiren OR Tekamlo OR Valturna OR Midimor OR Amiloride OR Norvasc OR Amlodipine OR Caduet OR Lotrel OR Tenormin OR Atenolol OR Tenoretic OR Edarbi OR Azilsartan OR Lotensin OR Benazepril OR Kerlone OR Betaxolol OR Zebeta OR Bisoprolol OR Atacand OR Candesartan OR Coreg OR Carvedilol OR Diuril OR Chlorothiazide OR Thalitone OR Chlorthalidone OR Clorpres OR Catapres OR Clonidine OR Cardizem OR diltiazem OR Cartia OR Dilacor OR Dilt OR Diltia OR Matzim OR Taztia OR Tiamate OR Tiazac OR Avapro OR irbesartan OR Dynacirc OR isradipine OR Trandate OR labetalol OR Prinivil OR lisinopril OR Zestril OR Cozaar OR losartan OR Zaroxloyn OR metolazone OR Lopressor OR metoprolol OR Toprol OR Univasc OR moexipril OR Corgard OR nadalol OR Bystolic OR nebivolol OR Cardene OR nicardipine OR Procardia OR nifedipine OR Sular OR nisoldipine OR Benicar OR olmesartan OR Levitol OR penbutolol OR Aceon OR perindopril OR Pindolol OR pindolol OR Minipress OR prazosin OR Inderal OR propranolol OR Accupril OR quinapril OR Altace OR ramipril OR Micardis OR telmisartan OR Demadex OR torsemide OR Mavik OR trandolapril OR Diovan OR valsartan OR Calan OR verapamil OR Covera OR Isoptin OR Verelan OR Antihypertensive OR antihypertensives OR Hypolipidemic OR hypolipidemics OR "Nicotinic Agonists" OR Heparin OR Warfarin OR anticoagulant OR anticoagulants OR bupropion)
#6	DE "Smoking Cessation" OR TI (smoking OR tobacco) OR AB (smoking OR tobacco) OR DE "Diets" OR DE "Aerobic Exercise" OR DE "Weightlifting" OR DE "Yoga" OR DE "Movement Therapy" OR DE "Physical Activity" OR DE "Exercise" OR DE "Behavior Therapy" OR DE "Aversion Therapy" OR DE "Conversion Therapy" OR DE "Dialectical Behavior Therapy" OR DE "Exposure Therapy" OR DE "Implosive Therapy" OR DE "Reciprocal Inhibition Therapy" OR DE "Response Cost" OR DE "Systematic Desensitization Therapy" OR DE "Cognitive Behavior Therapy" OR DE "Acceptance and Commitment Therapy" OR DE "Health Education" OR DE "Drug Education" OR DE "Sex Education" AND DE "Counseling" OR DE "Educational Counseling" OR DE "Group Counseling" OR DE "Microcounseling" OR DE "Peer Counseling" OR DE "Psychotherapeutic Counseling" OR DE "Family Therapy" OR DE "Disease Management" OR DE "Lifestyle Changes" OR DE "Treatment Compliance" OR DE "Relapse Prevention" OR DE "Motivational Interviewing" OR DE "Self Monitoring" OR DE "Weight Loss" OR TI (exercise OR "physical activity" OR diet OR diets OR "weight management" OR counsel* OR "cognitive behavioral therapy" OR "lifestyle modification" OR adher* OR "self-monitoring" OR "relapse prevention" OR "skills training" OR "motivational interviewing" OR educat*) OR AB (exercise OR "physical activity" OR diet OR diets OR "weight management" OR counsel* OR "cognitive behavioral therapy" OR "lifestyle modification" OR adher* OR "self-monitoring" OR "relapse prevention" OR "skills training" OR "motivational interviewing" OR educat*)
#7	DE "Social Support" OR TI (family OR peer) OR AB (family OR peer)
#8	TI (substitut* OR switch OR switched OR switching OR change OR changed OR changing OR replace OR replaced OR replacing OR replacement OR abandon*) AND AB (substitut* OR switch OR switched OR switching OR change OR changed OR changing OR replace OR replaced OR replacing OR replacement OR abandon*)

Set #	Terms
#9	#8 AND #3
#10	#5 OR #6 OR #7 OR #9
#11	#4 AND #10 Limiters - English; Methodology: TREATMENT OUTCOME/CLINICAL TRIAL

Grey Literature Searches

ClinicalTrials.gov (July 25, 2012)

Table A-17. ClinicalTrials.gov

Set #	Terms
Search terms	antipsychotic OR antipsychotics OR weight OR obesity OR obese OR overweight OR diabetes OR dyslipidemia OR hyperlipidemia OR cardiovascular OR hypertension
Condition	Schizophrenia OR bipolar disorder OR "serious mental illness" OR psychotic depression OR "severe mental illness" OR "severe psychiatric illness"
Intervention	behavioral OR drug OR drugs OR switch OR switching OR substitute OR substitution
Limits	Intervention studies, Adults/Seniors

Appendix B. Efficacy–Effectiveness Rating Form

<u>Directions</u>: For each article, rate the study along eight dimensions. For each dimension, consider whether, on balance, the study is most consistent with the definition of efficacy or effectiveness. Make your best judgment, but if the article does not give adequate information to make a determination, choose "unclear."

Table B-1. Efficacy–Effectiveness Rating Form

Dimension	Efficacy/Explanatory Trial	Effectiveness/Pragmatic Trial
1. Setting/practitioner expertise ☐ Efficacy ☐ Effectiveness ☐ Unclear	*Highly specialized setting:* Research clinic/ integrated MH-Gen Med Health **OR** referral population **OR** Academic medical Center **OR** restricted to practitioners with additional training in the intervention	*Reflects typical care setting:* Community settings (e.g. CMHC, PC) or full range of usual care settings **AND** practitioners do not have any special intervention training
2. Eligibility criteria ☐ Efficacy ☐ Effectiveness ☐ Unclear	*Captures narrow spectrum of SMI population:* Convenience sample **OR** sample selection criteria that excludes typical psychiatric comorbidities (e.g., mood or anxiety disorder), medical comorbidities (e.g., stable DM, HTN) or medications (e.g., antidepressants, mood stabilizers) **OR** those less likely to adhere to treatment (fail run-in period); **OR** small proportion of those evaluated are eligible (<25%)	*Captures full spectrum of SMI population:* Consecutive patients **OR** allows usual comorbidities and those less likely to be adherent, **AND** a high proportion of those evaluated are eligible
3. Health outcomes ☐ Efficacy ☐ Effectiveness ☐ Unclear	*Focus on intermediate outcomes:* Does not include clinical events (e.g., MI, stroke, major DM complications), physical function, mortality or health-related quality of life	*Clinically important outcomes included:* In the methods section, specifies ≥ 1 of the following outcomes: clinical events, mortality, physical function, or HRQOL
4. Study duration/clinically relevant intervention ☐ Efficacy ☐ Effectiveness ☐ Unclear	*Short duration/Fixed intervention:* Intervention duration and dose is fixed, **OR** outcomes are short-term only (<6 months)	*Longer duration/Flexible intervention:* Intervention dose or duration given to clinical endpoints or Intervention is flexible and responds to clinical status, **AND** outcomes are longer-term (≥ 6 months)
5. Assessment of adverse events ☐ Efficacy ☐ Effectiveness ☐ Unclear	*Adverse events are not measured/reported carefully:* Does not report discontinuation due to AE and ≥ 1 other predefined, important AE; **OR** measures are <u>not</u> obtained with a scale	*Adverse events are measured/reported carefully:* Reports discontinuation due to AE, and ≥ 1 other predefined, important AE; measures are obtained with a scale

Dimension	Efficacy/Explanatory Trial	Effectiveness/Pragmatic Trial
6. Adequate sample size for health outcomes ☐ Efficacy ☐ Effectiveness ☐ Unclear	*Inadequate/Unspecified sample size*: Sample size not given for clinical events, physical function, mortality or HRQOL	*Adequate sample size*: Sample size calculation given for clinical events, physical function, mortality or HRQOL
7. ITT analysis ☐ Efficacy ☐ Effectiveness ☐ Unclear	*No ITT analysis*: Completers analysis or excludes those with protocol deviations	*ITT analysis*: Follows intent-to-treat principle for analysis (includes all patients regardless of compliance, eligibility)
Study quality	Captured from quality rating tool	Captured from quality rating tool
Experimental domain		
8. Comparison intervention ☐ Efficacy ☐ Effectiveness ☐ Unclear	Comparison is placebo rather than the best alternative management strategy	Usual practice or the best alternative management strategy, offering practitioners considerable leeway in deciding how to apply it

Comments:

Appendix C. Data Abstraction Elements

Study Characteristics
- Study Identifiers
  - o Study Name or Acronym
  - o Last name of first author
- Additional Articles Used in This Abstraction
- Recruitment Dates (month and year)
  - o Start of recruitment
  - o End of recruitment
- Number of Sites
- Geographic Location (Select all that apply)
  - o US, Canada, UK, Europe, S. America, C. America, Asia, Africa, Australia/NZ, Not reported/Unclear, Other (specify)
- Funding Source (Select all that apply)
  - o Government, Private Foundation, Industry, Not reported/Unclear, Other (specify)
- Setting (Select all that apply)
  - o Outpatient mental health settings; Outpatient general medical settings; Community settings (e.g., community center, clubhouse); Integrated care setting (e.g., mental health and primary care provider work together to provide care to SMI population); Not reported; Other (specify)
- Study Inclusion and Exclusion Criteria
  - o Study Inclusion Criteria (Check all that apply)
    - Schizophrenia or schizoaffective disorder (or other related primary psychotic disorder: Psychotic D/O NOS, Delusional Disorder, Schizophreniform disorder, Brief psychotic disorder)
    - Bipolar disorder
    - Psychotic depression
    - No specified diagnosis but are classified as having SMI or SPMI
    - Taking an antipsychotic medication
    - Obese (BMI $\geq$ 30)
    - Overweight (BMI = 25-29.9)
    - Diabetes or elevated glucose
    - Hyperlipidemia or elevated lipids
    - Hypertension
    - Metabolic syndrome
    - Elevated CVD risk (mix or not specified by conditions above)
    - Age (specify)
    - None of the above
  - o Copy/paste inclusion criteria as reported in article
  - o Study Exclusion Criteria (Check all that apply)
    - Active substance abuse
    - Unstable psychiatric illness (acute illness)
    - Pregnant or breastfeeding
    - Participating in formal weight loss program
    - On additional medication other than study medications (specify)
    - Mental retardation

- - - Treatment refractory mental illness
    - Chronic medical condition (specify)
    - Unable to provide informed consent
    - Suicidality
    - Homicidality
    - Obese (BMI $\geq$ 30)
    - Overweight (BMI = 25-29.9)
    - Diabetes or elevated glucose
    - Hyperlipidemia or elevated lipids
    - Hypertension
    - Metabolic syndrome
    - Elevated CVD risk (mix or not specified by conditions above)
    - None of the above
  - Copy/paste exclusion criteria as reported in article
- Study Enrollment/Study Completion
  - N Assessed for eligibility
  - N Eligible
  - N Randomized
  - N Completed followup (most distal time point of the primary outcome)
- Comments

Population Characteristics – Record the following elements for Total Population, Intervention Arm 1, Comparator Arm 1, and Comparator Arm 2
- Number of patients
- Descriptive name for group
- Gender (N)
  - Female
  - Male
- Ethnicity (N)
  - Hispanic or Latino
  - No Hispanic or Latino
- Race (N)
  - American Indian or Alaskan Native
  - Asian
  - Black or African American
  - Native Hawaiian or other Pacific Islander
  - White
  - Multiracial
  - Other
  - Not reported
- Age
  - Mean
  - Median
  - SD
  - Min Age
  - Max Age
  - 25% IQR
  - 75% IQR

- o Categorical
- Education (specify units)
  - o Mean
  - o Median
  - o SD
  - o Categorical
- SMI Symptom severity for Schizophrenia
  - o Indicate Scale Used
    - Clinical Global Impression (CGI) scale for psychosis
    - Brief Psychiatric Rating Scale (BPRS)
    - Positive and Negative Syndrome Scale (PANSS)
    - Global Assessment of Functioning (GAF)
    - Other (specify)
  - o Mean
  - o Median
  - o SD
  - o 25% IQR
  - o 75% IQR
  - o Categorical
- SMI Symptom severity for Bipolar disorder
  - o Indicate Scale Used
    - Clinical Global Impression – Bipolar Version (CGI-BP)
    - Young Mania Rating Scale (YMRS)
    - Global Assessment of Functioning (GAF)
    - Other (specify)
  - o Mean
  - o Median
  - o SD
  - o 25% IQR
  - o 75% IQR
  - o Categorical
- SMI Symptom severity for Psychotic Depression
  - o Scales Used
    - Hamilton Rating Scale for Depression (HAM-D)
    - Montgomery-Asberg Depression Rating Scale (MADRS)
    - Other (specify)
  - o Mean
  - o Median
  - o SD
  - o 25% IQR
  - o 75% IQR
  - o Categorical
- Smoking Status (N)
  - o Non-Smoker
  - o Current Smoker
  - o Former Smoker
- Weight as BMI
  - o Mean

- Median
  - SD
  - 25% IQR
  - 75% IQR
  - Categorical
- Weight (indicate kg or lbs)
  - Mean
  - Median
  - SD
  - 25% IQR
  - 75% IQR
  - Categorical
- HbA1c (%)
  - Average
  - Variance
- Lipids
  - Total Cholesterol (mg/dl)
    - Average
    - Variance
  - LDL (mg/dl)
    - Average
    - Variance
- Blood Pressure
  - Systolic (mmHg)
    - Average
    - Variance
  - Diastolic (mmHg)
    - Average
    - Variance
- Number of patients classified as obese/overweight at baseline
- Number of patients classified as having Diabetes (type not specified) at baseline
- Number of patients classified as having Type 1 Diabetes at baseline
- Number of patients classified as having Type 2 Diabetes at baseline
- Number of patients classified as having Hyperlipidemia at baseline
- Number of patients classified as having Metabolic Syndrome at baseline
- Number of patients classified as having hypertension at baseline
- SMI classification (N)
  - Schizophrenia
  - Bipolar
  - Psychotic
  - Not Specified
- SMI medication use (N)
  - 1st Gen Antipsychotics
  - 2nd Gen Antipsychotics
  - Mood stabilizers
  - Antidepressants
  - Mixed or combination therapy
- Describe other relevant comorbid conditions

Intervention Characteristics
- Background Context of Interventions
- Intervention Arm – Indicate the target chronic medical illness for the intervention
  - Weight (obese or overweight at baseline)
  - Obesity prevention
  - Diabetes (not specified)
  - Type 1 Diabetes
  - Type 2 Diabetes
  - Hyperlipidemia
  - Hypertension
  - Multimodal cardiovascular disease
  - Other (specify)
- Intervention Components per Arm
  - For the Intervention Arm
    - Descriptive Name
    - Components (Check all that apply)
      - Patient-focused behavioral interventions for one condition of interest
        - Were drugs used in behavioral intervention? (Yes/No)
      - Pharmacological treatments for chronic medical condition
      - Antipsychotic medication switching
      - Multimodal lifestyle intervention targeting multiple CVD risk factors
        - Were drugs used in lifestyle intervention? (Yes/No)
  - For Comparator Arm 1 and Comparator Arm 2
    - Descriptive Name
    - Components (Check all that apply)
      - Usual
      - Enhanced usual care (please describe)
      - Attention control (please describe)
      - Placebo control
      - Patient focused behavioral interventions for one condition of interest
        - Were drugs used in behavioral intervention? (Yes/No)
      - Pharmacological treatments for chronic medical condition
      - Antipsychotic medication switching
      - Multimodal lifestyle intervention targeting multiple CVD risk factors
        - Were drugs used in lifestyle intervention? (Yes/No)
  - If 'Patient-focused behavioral interventions for one condition of interest' or 'Multimodal lifestyle intervention targeting multiple CVD risk factors' are selected, specify the following:
    - Patient-focused behavioral interventions for one condition of interest
      - Total planned contacts
      - Mean (SD) contacts delivered
      - Mode (check all that apply)
        - In person; Phone; Internet; Text messaging
          - Frequency of planned contact

- Theoretical orientation or health behavioral theory informing interventions (e.g., Health Belief Model, Social Cognitive Theory, Transtheoretical Model)
    - Not reported/No
    - Yes (specify)
- Therapeutic Model or orientation
    - Not reported/No
    - Cognitive Behavioral therapy (CBT)
    - Dialectic Behavioral Therapy (DBT)
    - Motivational Interviewing (MI)
    - Psychodynamic therapy
    - Behavioral Therapy
    - Cognitive Therapy
    - Problem-solving Therapy (PST)
    - Insight-oriented therapy
    - Interpersonal Psychotherapy (IPT)
    - Acceptance and Commitment Therapy (ACT)
    - Rational Emotive Behavior Therapy (REBT)
    - Relaxation
    - Emotion-focused therapy
    - Solution-focused therapy
    - Token economy
    - Social-skills training
    - Family therapy
    - Other (specify)
- Intervention delivered by (interventionist type)
    - NA
    - Not reported
    - Nurse
    - Behavioral health profession (e.g., social worker, psychologist)
    - Health educator
    - Peer support specialist
    - Peer educator (intervention provider has a current or past history of mental illness)
    - Nutritionist
    - Physical therapist
    - Physician
    - Other (specify)
- Level of training for interventionist
    - NA
    - Not reported
    - Describe level of training
- Are family members engaged in the intervention?
    - Yes
    - No
    - Unclear
- Content Covered

- Patient psychoeducational (education about mental illness provided to patient)
- Family psychoeducational (education about mental illness provided to family members)
- Chronic physical health condition education (e.g. diabetes education on prevalence and etiology)
- Diet/nutrition
- Physical activity/exercise
- Smoking cessation (e.g. behavioral strategies for quitting, NRT)
- SMI medication management/adherence
- Medical management for chronic physical health condition (e.g. insulin, statins)
- Other (specify)
- Not reported
- Strategies Used
  - Not reported
  - Problem solving skills
  - Goal setting (e.g. weight goals, minutes of physical activity a week)
  - Motivational techniques
  - Self-monitoring (e.g. getting on home scale for weight, glucose or BP monitoring)
  - Activity scheduling
  - Stress management techniques
  - Telemonitoring
  - Economic incentives
  - Personalized or tailored written communications for home use (e.g. personalized health plan)
  - Strategies to enhance social support
  - Homework assignments
  - Other (specify)
- Other non-patient directed strategies (i.e., organization or structural changes directed at providers or systems)
  - NA
  - Provider education (e.g. CME, clinical guideline)
  - Care management (e.g. nurse case manager)
  - Integration or co-location of care model
  - Other (describe)
- Description of intervention sufficient for replication?
  - Yes (e.g. manualized intervention)
  - No (insufficient details)
- If 'Pharmacological treatments for chronic medical condition' is selected, specify the following:
  - Pharmacological treatments for chronic medical condition
    - Psychotropic drug(s): Aripiprazole, Asenapine, Chlorpromazine, Glozapine, Haloperidol, Iloperidone, Loxapine, Molindone, Olanzapine, Olanzapine and Fluoxetine (Symbyax), Paliperidone,

Pimozide, Quetiapine, Risperidone, Thiothixene, Trifluoperazine, Ziprasidone
- o Dose range (mg/day)
- o Fixed dose (Yes/No)
- o Mean dose (mg/day)
- o Treatment duration (weeks)

- Weight loss drug(s): Orlistat, Metformin, Topiramate, Other (specify)
  - o Dose range (mg/day)
  - o Fixed dose (Yes/No)
  - o Mean dose (mg/day)
  - o Treatment duration (weeks)

- Diabetes drug(s): Bromocriptine, Colesevelam, Exenitide, Glimepiride, Glyburide, Insulin, Insulin aspart, Insulin detemir, Insulin glargine, Insulin glulisine, Insulin isophane, Insulin lispro, Linagliptin, Liraglutide, Metformin, Miglitol, Nateglinide, Pioglitazone, Pramlinitide, Repaglinide, Rosiglitazone, Saxagliptin, Sitagliptin
  - o Dose range (mg/day)
  - o Fixed dose (Yes/No)
  - o Mean dose (mg/day)
  - o Treatment duration (weeks)

- Hyperlipidemia drug(s): Atorvastatin, Atorvastatin/amlodipine, Cholestyramine, Colesevelam, Colestipol, Ezetimibe, Fenofibrate, Fluvastatin, Lovastatin, Pitavastatin, Pravastatin, Rosuvastatin, Simvastatin
  - o Dose range (mg/day)
  - o Fixed dose (Yes/No)
  - o Mean dose (mg/day)
  - o Treatment duration (weeks)

- Other drug for chronic medical condition: specify
  - o Dose range (mg/day)
  - o Fixed dose (Yes/No)
  - o Mean dose (mg/day)
  - o Treatment duration (weeks)

- o If 'Antipsychotic medication switching' is selected, specify the following:
  - ▪ Antipsychotic switch strategy
    - • Dose range (mg/day)
    - • Fixed dose (Ycs/No)
    - • Mean dose (mg/day)
    - • Treatment duration (weeks)
  - ▪ Current therapy
    - • Dose range (mg/day)
    - • Fixed dose (Yes/No)
    - • Mean dose (mg/day)
    - • Treatment duration (weeks)

- Comments

Outcomes

Record the following elements for Total Population, Intervention Arm 1, Comparator Arm 1, and Comparator Arm 2 as applicable

- Select the outcome reported on this form:
  - BMI
  - Weight in lbs
  - Weight in kilograms
  - HbA1c (%)
  - HBA1c (<7%)
  - Total Cholesterol (mg/dl)
  - LDL (mg/dl)
  - Systolic blood pressure (mm Hg)
  - Diastolic blood pressure (mm Hg)
  - Systolic blood pressure (<130 mm Hg)
  - Diastolic blood pressure (<80 mm Hg)
  - Smoking cessation
  - Framingham risk score
  - Other CVD summary risk score
  - Psychiatric symptom severity
  - All-cause mortality
  - CVD-only mortality
  - HRQOL/Physical function (specify in Details field)
  - Adverse event/ significant worsening of psychiatric status (as defined by the study author)
  - Adverse event/ Discontinuation due to adverse event or serious adverse event
  - Adverse event/Death
  - Adverse event/Hospitalization
  - Adverse event/other
  - Other potentially relevant outcome (specify)
- Is this a special population? (Yes/No)
  - If yes: Define special population
- Additional details describing outcome definition
- Time points abstracted
  - Time point closest to 3 months
  - Time point closest to 6 months
  - Most distal time point
- For each time point record the following elements as applicable
  - Specify actual timing of outcome
  - N Analyzed
  - Unadjusted Result
    - Mean
    - Median
    - Mean within group change
    - Mean between group change
    - Number of patients with outcome
    - % of patients with outcome
    - Events/denominator
    - Odds ratio

- - Hazard ratio
  - Relative risk
  - Other (specify)
  - Unadjusted Result Variability
    - Standard Error (SE)
    - Standard Deviation (SD)
    - Range
    - Other (specify)
  - Unadjusted Result, CI or IQR
    - 95% CI
    - Other % CI (specify)
    - IQR
  - Unadjusted Result, p-value between groups
  - Unadjusted Result, Reference group (for comparisons between groups)
  - Adjusted Result
    - Mean
    - Median
    - Mean within group change
    - Mean between group change
    - Number of patients with outcome
    - % of patients with outcome
    - Events/denominator
    - Odds ratio
    - Hazard ratio
    - Relative risk
    - Other (specify)
  - Adjusted Result Variability
    - Standard Error (SE)
    - Standard Deviation (SD)
    - Range
    - Other (specify)
  - Adjusted Result, CI or IQR
    - 95% CI
    - Other % CI (specify)
    - IQR
  - Adjusted Result, p-value between groups
  - Adjusted Result, Reference group (for comparison between groups)
- Indicate adjustments applied
- Was data reported for this outcome at any other time points? (Yes/No)
  - If Yes: List other time points
- Does the study report any subgroup analyses for this outcome? (Yes/No)
  - If Yes: Describe the subgroup analyses and summarize results
- Contact Study Author
  - Are there critical variables that have missing or confusing information such that we should contact the study authors for additional information? (Yes/No)
    - If Yes: List information needed
- Comments

Quality Assessment

- Selection Bias
    - Was the allocation sequence adequately generated? (Yes/No/Unclear)
    - Was the allocation adequately concealed? (Yes/No/Unclear)
    - Did the strategy for recruiting participants into the study remain the same across study groups? (Yes/No/Unclear)
    - Was there an absence of systematic differences observed in baseline characteristics and prognostic factors across the groups compared? If no, did the analysis control for differences? (Yes/No/Unclear)
- Performance Bias
    - Did researchers rule out any impact from a concurrent intervention or an unintended exposure (e.g., some members of control group get intervention), that might bias results? (Yes/No/Unclear)
    - Was execution of the intervention a close match for plans in the study protocol (i.e., no variation from the study protocol which could compromise conclusion of the study)? (Yes/No/Unclear)
- Attrition Bias
    - Was there a low rate of differential attrition (defined as less than 10% difference between groups)? (Yes/No/Unclear)
    - Was incomplete outcome data adequately addressed? (Yes/No/Unclear)
- Detection Bias
    - Were outcome assessors blind to treatment assignment of weight, laboratory measurements (e.g., LDL, HbA1c), and mortality? (Yes/No/Unclear)
    - Were outcome assessors blind to treatment assignment of all other outcomes (psychiatric symptom severity, adverse effects, HRQL)? (Yes/No/Unclear)
    - Are the inclusion/exclusion criteria measured using reliable and valid measures, implemented consistently across groups? (Yes/No/Unclear)
    - Are primary outcomes assessed using reliable and valid measures, implemented consistently across groups? (Yes/No/Unclear)
- Reporting Bias
    - Are the potential outcomes pre-specified by the researchers? Are all pre-specified outcomes reported? (Yes/No/Unclear)
- Conflict of Interest
    - Was there the absence of potential important conflict of interest? (Yes/No/Unclear)
- Study ratings:
    - A "Good" study has the least bias, and results are considered valid. A good study has a clear description of the population, setting, interventions, and comparison groups; uses a valid approach to allocate patients to alternative treatments; has a low dropout rate; and uses appropriate means to prevent bias, measure outcomes, and analyze and report results.
    - A "Fair" study is susceptible to some bias but probably not enough to invalidate the results. The study may be missing information, making it difficult to assess limitations and potential problems. As the fair-quality category is broad, studies with this rating vary in their strengths and weaknesses. The results of some fair-quality studies are possibly valid, while others are probably valid.
    - A "Poor" rating indicates significant bias that may invalidate the results. These studies have serious errors in design, analysis, or reporting; have large amounts of missing information; or have discrepancies in reporting. The results of a poor-quality

study are at least as likely to reflect flaws in the study design as to indicate true differences between the compared interventions.

- Study rating for weight, laboratory measurements (e.g., LDL, HbA1c), and mortality
  - Good
  - Fair
  - Poor
  - No outcomes of this type reported
  - If the study is rated as 'Fair' or 'Poor,' provide rationale for decision
- Study rating for all other outcomes (i.e., Adverse effects, HRQL, psychiatric symptom severity)
  - Good
  - Fair
  - Poor
  - No outcomes of this type reported
  - If the study is rated as 'Fair' or 'Poor,' provide rationale for decision
- Comments

Applicability

- Population
  - Is the study eligibility criteria narrowly defined such that it excludes those with comorbidities common in the SMI population? (Yes/No/Unclear)
- Interventions
  - Is the intervention team highly selected or at a level of training and proficiency not widely available? (Yes/No/Unclear)
- Comparator
  - Was the comparator composed of a substandard therapy not used in usual care of condition (e.g., statin for lipids, brief counseling for smoking)? (Yes/No/Unclear)
- Outcomes
  - Were only short-term outcomes (<6 months) measured? (Yes/No/Unclear)
- Setting
  - Were the majority of patients recruited in the US? (Yes/No/Unclear)

Efficacy-Effectiveness Rating

- Setting/Practitioner expertise (Efficacy/Effectiveness/Unclear)
  - Efficacy/Explanatory Trial
    - Highly specialized setting: Research clinic/ integrated MH-Gen Med Health OR referral population OR Academic medical Center OR restricted to practitioners with additional training in the intervention
  - Effectiveness/Pragmatic Trial
    - Reflects typical care setting: Community settings (e.g. CMHC, PC) or full range of usual care settings AND practitioners do not have any special intervention training
- Eligibility criteria (Efficacy/Effectiveness/Unclear)
  - Efficacy/Explanatory Trial
    - Captures narrow spectrum of SMI population: Convenience sample OR sample selection criteria that excludes typical psychiatric comorbidities (e.g., mood or anxiety disorder), medical comorbidities (e.g., stable DM, HTN) or medications (e.g., antidepressants, mood stabilizers) OR those less likely to

adhere to treatment (fail run-in period); OR small proportion of those evaluated are eligible (<25%)
- o Effectiveness/Pragmatic Trial
  - ▪ Captures full spectrum of SMI population: Consecutive patients OR allows usual comorbidities and those less likely to be adherent, AND a high proportion of those evaluated are eligible
- Health Outcomes (Efficacy/Effectiveness/Unclear)
  - o Efficacy/Explanatory Trial
    - ▪ Focus on intermediate outcomes: Does not include clinical events (e.g., MI, stroke, major DM complications), physical function, mortality or health-related quality of life
  - o Effectiveness/Pragmatic Trial
    - ▪ Clinically important outcomes included: In the methods section, specifies ≥ 1 of the following outcomes: clinical events, mortality, physical function, or HRQOL
- Study Duration/clinically relevant intervention (Efficacy/Effectiveness/Unclear)
  - o Efficacy/Explanatory Trial
    - ▪ Short duration/Fixed intervention: Intervention duration and dose is fixed, OR outcomes are short-term only (<6 months)
  - o Effectiveness/Pragmatic Trial
    - ▪ Longer duration/Flexible intervention: Intervention dose or duration given to clinical endpoints or Intervention is flexible and responds to clinical status, AND outcomes are longer-term (≥ 6 months)
- Assessment of adverse events (Efficacy/Effectiveness/Unclear)
  - o Efficacy/Explanatory Trial
    - ▪ Adverse events are not measured/reported carefully: Does not report discontinuation due to AE and ≥ 1 other predefined, important AE; OR measures are not obtained with a scale.
  - o Effectiveness/Pragmatic Trial
    - ▪ Adverse events are measured/reported carefully: Reports discontinuation due to AE, and ≥ 1 other predefined, important AE; measures are obtained with a scale.
- Adequate sample size for health outcomes (Efficacy/Effectiveness/Unclear)
  - o Efficacy/Explanatory Trial
    - ▪ Inadequate/Unspecified sample size: Sample size not given for clinical events, physical function, mortality or HRQOL
  - o Effectiveness/Pragmatic Trial
    - ▪ Adequate sample size: Sample size calculation given clinical events, physical function, mortality or HRQOL
- ITT analysis (Efficacy/Effectiveness/Unclear)
  - o Efficacy/Explanatory Trial
    - ▪ No ITT analysis: Completers analysis or excludes those with protocol deviations.
  - o Effectiveness/Pragmatic Trial
    - ▪ ITT analysis: Follows intent-to-treat principle for analysis (includes all patients regardless of compliance, eligibility)
- Study quality: Captured from quality rating tool
- Experimental domain - Comparison intervention (Efficacy/Effectiveness/Unclear)

- o Efficacy/Explanatory Trial
  - ▪ Comparison is placebo rather than the best alternative management strategy
- o Effectiveness/Pragmatic Trial
  - ▪ Usual practice or the best alternative management strategy, offering practitioners considerable leeway in deciding how to apply it.
- Comments

Appendix D. Included Studies

Table D-1 lists all included studies by primary article in alphabetical order, companion article (if applicable), and study designation (if applicable). Full bibliographic citations follow the table.

Table D-1. Studies included in SMI comparative effectiveness review

Primary Article	Companion Article	Study Designation
Alvarez-Jimenez, 2006[1]	Alvarez-Jimenez, 2010[2]	NA
Assuncao, 2006[3]	NA	NA
Atmaca, 2003[4]	NA	NA
Atmaca, 2004[5]	NA	NA
Ball, 2011[6]	NA	NA
Borba, 2011[7]	NA	NA
Brar, 2005[8]	NA	NA
Brown, 2011[9]	NA	NA
Bustillo, 2003[10]	NA	NA
Carrizo, 2009[11]	Fernandez, 2010[12]	NA
Cavazzoni, 2003[13]	NA	NA
Deberdt, 2008[14]	NA	NA
Elmslie, 2006[15]	NA	NA
Evans, 2005[16]	NA	NA
Fleischhacker, 2010[17]	NA	NA
Forsberg, 2008[18]	NA	NA
Gillhoff, 2010[19]	NA	NA
Graham, 2005[20]	NA	NA
Hoffmann, 2012[21]	NA	NA
Kwon, 2006[22]	NA	NA
Karagianis, 2009[23]	Karagianis, 2010[24]	PLATYPUS
Khazaal, 2007[25]	NA	NA
Littrell, 2003[26]	NA	NA
Mauri, 2008[27]	NA	NA
McDonnell, 2011[28]	NA	NA
McElroy, 2012[29]	NA	NA
McKibbin, 2006[30]	Leutwyler, 2010[31] McKibbin, 2010[32]	Diabetes Awareness and Rehabilitation Training (DART)
Narula, 2010[33]	NA	NA
Newcomer, 2008[34]	NA	NA
Nickel, 2005[35]	NA	NA

Primary Article	Companion Article	Study Designation
Skrinar, 2005[36]	NA	NA
Stroup, 2011[37]	NA	Comparison of Antipsychotics for Metabolic Problems (CAMP)
Wang 2012[38]	NA	NA
Wu, 2008[39]	NA	NA
Wu, 2012[40]	NA	NA

Abbreviations: NA=not applicable; SMI-serious mental illness

References Cited in Appendix D

1. Alvarez-Jimenez M, Gonzalez-Blanch C, Vazquez-Barquero JL, et al. Attenuation of antipsychotic-induced weight gain with early behavioral intervention in drug-naive first-episode psychosis patients: A randomized controlled trial. J Clin Psychiatry. 2006;67(8):1253-60. PMID: 16965204.

2. Alvarez-Jimenez M, Martinez-Garcia O, Perez-Iglesias R, et al. Prevention of antipsychotic-induced weight gain with early behavioural intervention in first-episode psychosis: 2-year results of a randomized controlled trial. Schizophr Res. 2010;116(1):16-9. PMID: 19896336.

3. Assuncao SS, Ruschel SI, Rosa Lde C, et al. Weight gain management in patients with schizophrenia during treatment with olanzapine in association with nizatidine. Rev Bras Psiquiatr. 2006;28(4):270-6. PMID: 17242805.

4. Atmaca M, Kuloglu M, Tezcan E, et al. Nizatidine treatment and its relationship with leptin levels in patients with olanzapine-induced weight gain. Hum Psychopharmacol. 2003;18(6):457-61. PMID: 12923824.

5. Atmaca M, Kuloglu M, Tezcan E, et al. Nizatidine for the treatment of patients with quetiapine-induced weight gain. Hum Psychopharmacol. 2004;19(1):37-40. PMID: 14716710.

6. Ball MP, Warren KR, Feldman S, et al. Placebo-controlled trial of atomoxetine for weight reduction in people with schizophrenia treated with clozapine or olanzapine. Clin Schizophr Relat Psychoses. 2011;5(1):17-25. PMID: 21459735.

7. Borba CP, Fan X, Copeland PM, et al. Placebo-controlled pilot study of ramelteon for adiposity and lipids in patients with schizophrenia. J Clin Psychopharmacol. 2011;31(5):653-8. PMID: 21869685.

8. Brar JS, Ganguli R, Pandina G, et al. Effects of behavioral therapy on weight loss in overweight and obese patients with schizophrenia or schizoaffective disorder. J Clin Psychiatry. 2005;66(2):205-12. PMID: 15705006.

9. Brown C, Goetz J, Hamera E. Weight loss intervention for people with serious mental illness: a randomized controlled trial of the RENEW program. Psychiatr Serv. 2011;62(7):800-2. PMID: 21724796.

10. Bustillo JR, Lauriello J, Parker K, et al. Treatment of weight gain with fluoxetine in olanzapine-treated schizophrenic outpatients. Neuropsychopharmacology. 2003;28(3):527-9. PMID: 12629532.

11. Carrizo E, Fernandez V, Connell L, et al. Extended release metformin for metabolic control assistance during prolonged clozapine administration: a 14 week, double-blind, parallel group, placebo-controlled study. Schizophr Res. 2009;113(1):19-26. PMID: 19515536.

12. Fernandez E, Carrizo E, Fernandez V, et al. Polymorphisms of the LEP- and LEPR genes, metabolic profile after prolonged clozapine administration and response to the antidiabetic metformin. Schizophr Res. 2010;121(1-3):213-7. PMID: 20591628.

13. Cavazzoni P, Tanaka Y, Roychowdhury SM, et al. Nizatidine for prevention of weight gain

with olanzapine: a double-blind placebo-controlled trial. Eur Neuropsychopharmacol. 2003;13(2):81-5. PMID: 12650950.

14. Deberdt W, Lipkovich I, Heinloth AN, et al. Double-blind, randomized trial comparing efficacy and safety of continuing olanzapine versus switching to quetiapine in overweight or obese patients with schizophrenia or schizoaffective disorder. Ther Clin Risk Manag. 2008;4(4):713-20. PMID: 19209252.

15. Elmslie JL, Porter RJ, Joyce PR, et al. Carnitine does not improve weight loss outcomes in valproate-treated bipolar patients consuming an energy-restricted, low-fat diet. Bipolar Disord. 2006;8(5 Pt 1):503-7. PMID: 17042889.

16. Evans S, Newton R, Higgins S. Nutritional intervention to prevent weight gain in patients commenced on olanzapine: a randomized controlled trial. Aust N Z J Psychiatry. 2005;39(6):479-86. PMID: 15943650.

17. Fleischhacker WW, Heikkinen ME, Olie JP, et al. Effects of adjunctive treatment with aripiprazole on body weight and clinical efficacy in schizophrenia patients treated with clozapine: a randomized, double-blind, placebo-controlled trial. Int J Neuropsychopharmacol. 2010;13(8):1115-25. PMID: 20459883.

18. Forsberg KA, Bjorkman T, Sandman PO, et al. Physical health--a cluster randomized controlled lifestyle intervention among persons with a psychiatric disability and their staff. Nord J Psychiatry. 2008;62(6):486-95 PMID: 18843564.

19. Gillhoff K, Gaab J, Emini L, et al. Effects of a multimodal lifestyle intervention on body mass index in patients with bipolar disorder: a randomized controlled trial. Prim Care Companion J Clin Psychiatry. 2010;12(5). PMID: 21274359.

20. Graham KA, Gu H, Lieberman JA, et al. Double-blind, placebo-controlled investigation of amantadine for weight loss in subjects who gained weight with olanzapine. Am J Psychiatry. 2005;162(9):1744-6. PMID: 16135638.

21. Hoffmann VP, Case M, Jacobson JG. Assessment of treatment algorithms including amantadine, metformin, and zonisamide for the prevention of weight gain with olanzapine: a randomized controlled open-label study. J Clin Psychiatry. 2012;73(2):216-23. PMID: 21672497.

22. Kwon JS, Choi JS, Bahk WM, et al. Weight management program for treatment-emergent weight gain in olanzapine-treated patients with schizophrenia or schizoaffective disorder: A 12-week randomized controlled clinical trial. J Clin Psychiatry. 2006;67(4):547-53. PMID: 16669719.

23. Karagianis J, Grossman L, Landry J, et al. A randomized controlled trial of the effect of sublingual orally disintegrating olanzapine versus oral olanzapine on body mass index: the PLATYPUS Study. Schizophr Res. 2009;113(1):41-8. PMID: 19535229.

24. Karagianis J, Landry J, Hoffmann VP, et al. An exploratory analysis of factors associated with weight change in a 16-week trial of oral vs. orally disintegrating olanzapine: the PLATYPUS study. Int J Clin Pract. 2010;64(11):1520-9. PMID: 20846199.

25. Khazaal Y, Fresard E, Rabia S, et al. Cognitive behavioural therapy for weight gain associated with antipsychotic drugs. Schizophr Res. 2007;91(1-3):169-77. PMID: 17306507.

26. Littrell KH, Hilligoss NM, Kirshner CD, et al. The effects of an educational intervention on antipsychotic-induced weight gain. J Nurs Scholarsh. 2003;35(3):237-41. PMID: 14562491.

27. Mauri M, Simoncini M, Castrogiovanni S, et al. A psychoeducational program for weight loss in patients who have experienced weight gain during antipsychotic treatment with olanzapine. Pharmacopsychiatry. 2008;41(1):17-23. PMID: 18203047.

28. McDonnell DP, Kryzhanovskaya LA, Zhao F, et al. Comparison of metabolic changes in patients with schizophrenia during randomized treatment with intramuscular olanzapine long-acting injection versus oral olanzapine. Hum Psychopharmacol. 2011;26(6):422-433. PMID: 21823172.

29. McElroy SL, Winstanley E, Mori N, et al. A randomized, placebo-controlled study of zonisamide to prevent olanzapine-associated weight gain. J Clin Psychopharmacol. 2012;32(2):165-72. PMID: 22367654.

30. McKibbin CL, Patterson TL, Norman G, et al. A lifestyle intervention for older schizophrenia patients with diabetes mellitus: a randomized

controlled trial. Schizophr Res. 2006;86(1-3):36-44. PMID: 16842977.

31. Leutwyler HC, Wallhagen M, McKibbin C. The impact of symptomatology on response to a health promoting intervention among older adults with schizophrenia. Diabetes Educ. 2010;36(6):945-55. PMID: 21119068.

32. McKibbin CL, Golshan S, Griver K, et al. A healthy lifestyle intervention for middle-aged and older schizophrenia patients with diabetes mellitus: a 6-month follow-up analysis. Schizophr Res. 2010;121(1-3):203-6. PMID: 20434886.

33. Narula PK, Rehan HS, Unni KE, et al. Topiramate for prevention of olanzapine associated weight gain and metabolic dysfunction in schizophrenia: a double-blind, placebo-controlled trial. Schizophr Res. 2010;118(1-3):218-23. PMID: 20207521.

34. Newcomer JW, Campos JA, Marcus RN, et al. A multicenter, randomized, double-blind study of the effects of aripiprazole in overweight subjects with schizophrenia or schizoaffective disorder switched from olanzapine. J Clin Psychiatry. 2008;69(7):1046-56. PMID: 18605811.

35. Nickel MK, Nickel C, Muehlbacher M, et al. Influence of topiramate on olanzapine-related adiposity in women: a random, double-blind, placebo-controlled study. J Clin Psychopharmacol. 2005;25(3):211-7. PMID: 15876898.

36. Skrinar GS, Huxley NA, Hutchinson DS, et al. The role of a fitness intervention on people with serious psychiatric disabilities. Psychiatr Rehabil J. 2005;29(2):122-7. PMID: 16268007.

37. Stroup TS, McEvoy JP, Ring KD, et al. A randomized trial examining the effectiveness of switching from olanzapine, quetiapine, or risperidone to aripiprazole to reduce metabolic risk: comparison of antipsychotics for metabolic problems (CAMP). Am J Psychiatry. 2011;168(9):947-56. PMID: 21768610.

38. Wang M, Tong JH, Zhu G, et al. Metformin for treatment of antipsychotic-induced weight gain: a randomized, placebo-controlled study. Schizophr Res. 2012;138(1):54-7. PMID: 22398127.

39. Wu RR, Zhao JP, Jin H, et al. Lifestyle intervention and metformin for treatment of antipsychotic-induced weight gain: a randomized controlled trial. JAMA. 2008;299(2):185-93. PMID: 18182600.

40. Wu RR, Jin H, Gao K, et al. Metformin for Treatment of Antipsychotic-Induced Amenorrhea and Weight Gain in Women With First-Episode Schizophrenia: A Double-Blind, Randomized, Placebo-Controlled Study. Am J Psychiatry. 2012;169(8):813-21. PMID: 22711171.

Appendix E. Excluded Studies

All studies listed below were reviewed in their full-text version and excluded for the reason shown in bold. Reasons for exclusion signify only the usefulness of the articles for this study and are not intended as criticisms of the articles.

Full text not available

Kostulski A, Rabe-Jablonska J. Effect of antipsychotic drugs on weight gain and metabolic disorders in schizophrenic patients.

Published prior to 1980

Gallant DM, Bishop MP, Schuchs V. A clinical trial of an oral hypoglycemic agent in chronic schizophrenic patients. Curr Ther Res Clin Exp. 1963;5:628-9. PMID: 14084034.

Harmatz MG, Lapuc P. Behavior modification of overeating in a psychiatric population. J Consult Clin Psychol. 1968;32(5):583-7. PMID: 5743317.

Modell W, Hussar AE. Failure of dextroamphetamine sulfate to influence eating and sleeping patterns in obese schizophrenic patients: clinical and pharmacological significance. JAMA. 1965;193:275-8. PMID: 14310348.

Sletten IW, Ognjanov V, Menendez S, et al. Weight reduction with chlorphenetermine and phenmetrazine in obese psychiatric patients during chlorpromazine therapy. Curr Ther Res Clin Exp. 1967;9(11):570-5. PMID: 4965506.

Non-English language

Lopez-Mato A, Rovner J, Illa G, et al. [Randomized, open label study on the use of ranitidine at different doses for the management of weight gain associated with olanzapine administration]. Vertex. 2003;14(52):85-96. PMID: 12883589.

Wang B, GP D. Behavioural intervention for antipsychotic caused weight gain.. Medical Journal of Chinese People's Health 2008;20(9):2117-8.

Not a full publication (abstract only)

Alvarez-Jimenez M. Tackling the physical consequences of psychosis and its treatment. Early Interv Psychiatry. 2010;4:17.

Firestone L, Ames D, Aragaki DLR, et al. Efficacy and safety of a lifestyle balance program for antipsychotic medication associated obesity. PM and R 2011;3(10 SUPPL. 1):S258-S259.

Ganguli R and Brar JS. Behavioural intervention for weight loss in schizophrenia: An RCT with active controls. Indian Journal of Psychiatry 2011;53(5 SUPPL. 1):S44.

Ginsberg DL. Add-on sibutramine for olanzapine-induced weight gain. Primary Psychiatry. 2004;11(7):24.

Greil W, Gillhoff K, Emini L, et al. Effects of a multimodal lifestyle intervention on body mass index in patients with bipolar disorder-a randomized controlled trial. Int Clin Psychopharmacol. 2011;26:e2.

Lieberman J, Jarskog LF, Hamer R, et al. Metformin for obesity and metabolic abnormalities in schizophrenia. Neuropsychopharmacology 2010;35 SUPPL. 1:S225-S226.

Lu RB and Lee SY. Add-on memantine to valproate treatment increase HDL in recently depressed patients with bipolar II disorder-a placebo-controlled 12-week study. Bipolar Disorders 2012;14 SUPPL. 1:99.

Newcomer J, Loebel A, Pikalov A, et al. Impact of lurasidone and olanzapine on framingham ten-year coronary heart disease risk estimate in schizophrenia. Neuropsychopharmacology 2010;35 SUPPL. 1:S334-S335.

Ratliff JC, Palmese LB, Tonizzo KM, et al. Pilot trial of contingency management for the treatment of antipsychotic-induced weight gain. Obesity 2011;19 SUPPL. 1:S99-S100.

Scheewe T, Kroes A, Takken T, et al. Effect of cardiovascular exercise on mental and physical health in patients with schizophrenia. European Archives of Psychiatry and Clinical Neuroscience 2011;261 SUPPL. 1:S97.

Slavkovic V, Tosic Golubovic S, Zikic O, et al. The influence of antipsychotics on the occurrence of the metabolic syndrome in schizophrenic patients. Eur Neuropsychopharmacol. 2011;21:S474-S475.

Stroup TS, Hamer RM, Ray N, et al. The effect of switching from olanzapine, quetiapine,or risperidone to aripiprazole on risk of cardiovascular disease: Results from the comparison of antipsychotics for metabolic problems (CAMP) study. Neuropsychopharmacology 2011;36 SUPPL. 1:S174.

Stroup TS, Hamer RM, Ray N, et al. The effect of switching from olanzapine, quetiapine, or risperidone to aripiprazole on risk of cardiovascular disease: Results from the comparison of antipsychotics for metabolic problems (CAMP) study. Neuropsychopharmacology 2011;36 SUPPL. 1:S424-S425.

Tek C, Ratliff JC, Reutenauer EL, et al. Naltrexone for antipsychotic-induced weight gain in women with schizophrenia. Biol Psychiatry. 2011;69(9):283S.

Tek C, Ratliff JC, Reutenauer EL, et al. Low-dose naltrexone for antipsychotic-induced weight gain in women with schizophrenia. Obesity 2011;19 SUPPL. 1:S181.

Not original peer-reviewed research paper

Baptista T, Beaulieu S. Body weight gain, insulin, and leptin in olanzapine-treated patients. J Clin Psychiatry. 2001;62(11):902-4. PMID: 11775052.

Casagrande SS, Jerome GJ, Dalcin AT, et al. Randomized trial of achieving healthy lifestyles in psychiatric rehabilitation: the ACHIEVE trial. BMC Psychiatry. 2010;10:108. PMID: 21144025.

Cohen D. Diabetes mellitus during olanzapine and quetiapine treatment in Japan. J Clin Psychiatry. 2005;66(2):265-6; author reply 266-7. PMID: 15705015

Dursun SM, Devarajan S. Clozapine weight gain, plus topiramate weight loss. Can J Psychiatry. 2000;45(2):198. PMID: 10742883.

Kim JH, Yim SJ, Nam JH. A 12-week, randomized, open-label, parallel-group trial of topiramate in limiting weight gain during olanzapine treatment in patients with schizophrenia. Schizophr Res. 2006;82(1):115-117.

Lessig MC, Shapira NA, Murphy TK. Topiramate for reversing atypical antipsychotic weight gain. J Am Acad Child Adolesc Psychiatry. 2001;40(12):1364. PMID: 11765278.

Levy E, Margolese HC, Chouinard G. Topiramate produced weight loss following olanzapine-induced weight gain in schizophrenia. J Clin Psychiatry. 2002;63(11):1045. PMID: 12469686.

Pavlovic ZM. Orlistat in the treatment of clozapine-induced hyperglycemia and weight gain. Eur Psychiatry. 2005;20(7):520. PMID: 16275033.

Post RM, Altshuler LL, Frye MA, et al. New findings from the Bipolar Collaborative Network: clinical implications for therapeutics. Curr Psychiatry Rep. 2006;8(6):489-97. PMID: 17162830.

Praharaj SK, Jana AK, Goyal N, et al. Metformin for olanzapine-induced weight gain: a systematic review and meta-analysis. Br J Clin Pharmacol. 2011;71(3):377-82. PMID: 21284696.

Not a randomized trial of 20 or more

Alptekin K, Hafez J, Brook S, et al. Efficacy and tolerability of switching to ziprasidone from olanzapine, risperidone or haloperidol: an international, multicenter study. Int Clin Psychopharmacol. 2009;24(5):229-38. PMID: 19531959.

Anghelescu I, Klawe C, Benkert O. Orlistat in the treatment of psychopharmacologically induced weight gain. J Clin Psychopharmacol. 2000;20(6):716-7. PMID: 11106155.

Arranz B, San L, Duenas RM, et al. Lower weight gain with the orally disintegrating olanzapine than with standard tablets in first-episode never treated psychotic patients. Hum Psychopharmacol. 2007;22(1):11-5. PMID: 17191265.

Bahk WM, Lee KU, Chae JH, et al. Open label study of the effect of amantadine on weight gain induced by olanzapine. Psychiatry Clin Neurosci. 2004;58(2):163-7. PMID: 15009821.

Baptista T, Hernandez L, Prieto LA, et al. Metformin in obesity associated with antipsychotic drug administration: a pilot study. J Clin Psychiatry. 2001;62(8):653-5. PMID: 11561940.

Bobo WV, Jayathilake K, Lee MA, et al. Changes in weight and body mass index during treatment with melperone, clozapine and typical neuroleptics. Psychiatry Res. 2010;176(2-3):114-9. PMID: 20199813.

Bradshaw T, Lovell K, Bee P, et al. The development and evaluation of a complex health education intervention for adults with a diagnosis of schizophrenia. J Psychiatr Ment Health Nurs. 2010;17(6):473-86. PMID: 20633074.

Brown C, Goetz J, Van Sciver A, et al. A psychiatric rehabilitation approach to weight loss. Psychiatr Rehabil J. 2006;29(4):267-73. PMID: 16689037.

Chawla B, Luxton-Andrew H. Long-term weight loss observed with olanzapine orally disintegrating tablets in overweight patients with chronic schizophrenia. A 1 year open-label, prospective trial. Hum Psychopharmacol. 2008;23(3):211-6. PMID: 18219624.

Colombo GL, Caruggi M, Di Matteo S, et al. An economic evaluation of aripiprazole vs olanzapine adapted to the Italian setting using outcomes of metabolic syndrome and risk for diabetes in patients with schizophrenia. Neuropsychiatr Dis Treat. 2008;4(5):967-76. PMID: 19183788.

Cosway R, Strachan MW, Dougall A, et al. Cognitive function and information processing in type 2 diabetes. Diabet Med. 2001;18(10):803-10. PMID: 11678970.

Faries DE, Ascher-Svanum H, Nyhuis AW, et al. Switching from risperidone to olanzapine in a one-year, randomized, open-label effectiveness study of schizophrenia. Curr Med Res Opin. 2008;24(5):1399-405. PMID: 18397549.

Gupta S, Droney T, Al-Samarrai S, et al. Olanzapine: weight gain and therapeutic efficacy. J Clin Psychopharmacol. 1999;19(3):273-5. PMID: 10350036.

Gupta S, Masand PS, Virk S, et al. Weight decline in patients switching from olanzapine to quetiapine. Schizophr Res. 2004;70(1):57-62.

Heggelund J, Nilsberg GE, Hoff J, et al. Effects of high aerobic intensity training in patients with schizophrenia: a controlled trial. Nord J Psychiatry. 2011;65(4):269-75. PMID: 21332297.

Henderson DC, Fan X, Copeland PM, et al. Aripiprazole added to overweight and obese olanzapine-treated schizophrenia patients. J Clin Psychopharmacol. 2009;29(2):165-9. PMID: 19512978.

Henderson DC, Fan X, Copeland PM, et al. Ziprasidone as an adjuvant for clozapine- or olanzapine-associated medical morbidity in chronic schizophrenia. Hum Psychopharmacol. 2009;24(3):225-32. PMID: 19283774.

Henderson DC, Fan X, Sharma B, et al. A double-blind, placebo-controlled trial of rosiglitazone for clozapine-induced glucose metabolism impairment in patients with schizophrenia. Acta Psychiatr Scand. 2009;119(6):457-65. PMID: 19183127.

Idomje OB, Festus OO, Akpamu U, et al. A comparative study of the effects of clozapine and risperidone monotherapy on lipid profile in Nigerian patients with schizophrenia. International Journal of Pharmacology 2012;8(3):170-176. PMID: 2012183764.

Iglesias-Garcia C, Toimil-Iglesias A and Alonso-Villa MJ. Pilot study of the efficacy of an educational programme to reduce weight, on overweight and obese patients with chronic stable schizophrenia. J Psychiatr Ment Health Nurs. 2010;17(9):849-51. PMID: 21077409.

Jean-Baptiste M, Tek C, Liskov E, et al. A pilot study of a weight management program with food provision in schizophrenia. Schizophr Res. 2007;96(1-3):198-205. PMID: 17628437.

Karayal ON, Glue P, Bachinsky M, et al. Switching from quetiapine to ziprasidone: a sixteen-week, open-label, multicenter study evaluating the effectiveness and safety of ziprasidone in outpatient subjects with schizophrenia or schizoaffective disorder. J Psychiatr Pract. 2011;17(2):100-9. PMID: 21430488.

Kim S-W, Shin I-S, Kim J-M, et al. Effectiveness of switching to aripiprazole from atypical antipsychotics in patients with schizophrenia. Clin Neuropharmacol. 2009;32(5):243-249.

Kline NS, Blair J, Cooper TB, et al. A controlled sevn year study of endocrine and other indices in drug treated chronic schizophrenics. Acta Psychiatr Scand Suppl. 1968;206:7-75. PMID: 4890732.

Larmo I, de Nayer A, Windhager E, et al. Efficacy and tolerability of quetiapine in patients with schizophrenia who switched from haloperidol, olanzapine or risperidone. Hum Psychopharmacol. 2005;20(8):573-81. PMID: 16175656.

McEvoy J, Freudenreich O, McGee M, et al. Clozapine decreases smoking in patients with chronic schizophrenia. Biol Psychiatry. 1995;37(8):550-2. PMID: 7619979.

Porsdal V, Beal C, Kleivenes OK, et al. The Scandinavian Solutions for Wellness study - a two-arm observational study on the effectiveness of lifestyle intervention on subjective well-being and weight among persons with psychiatric disorders. BMC Psychiatry. 2010;10:42. PMID: 20537122.

Poulin MJ, Chaput JP, Simard V, et al. Management of antipsychotic-induced weight gain: prospective naturalistic study of the effectiveness of a supervised exercise programme. Aust N Z J Psychiatry. 2007;41(12):980-9. PMID: 17999270.

Sajatovic M, Dawson NV, Perzynski AT, et al. Best practices: Optimizing care for people with serious mental illness and comorbid diabetes. Psychiatr Serv. 2011;62(9):1001-3. PMID: 21885575.

Sajatovic M, Dawson NV, Perzynski AT, et al. Best practices: Optimizing care for people with serious mental illness and comorbid diabetes. Psychiatr Serv 2011;62(9):1001-3. PMID: 21885575.

Sato Y, Yasui-Furukori N, Furukori H, et al. A crossover study on the glucose metabolism between treatment with olanzapine and risperidone in schizophrenic patients. Exp Clin Psychopharmacol. 2010;18(5):445-50. PMID: 20939648.

Skouroliakou M, Giannopoulou I, Kostara C, et al. Effects of a nutritional intervention in obese postmenopausal women on atypical antipsychotics. Maturitas. 2010;67(2):166-70. PMID: 20605075.

Skouroliakou M, Giannopoulou I, Kostara C, et al. Effects of nutritional intervention on body weight and body composition of obese psychiatric patients taking olanzapine. Nutrition. 2009;25(7-8):729-35. PMID: 19286349.

Takahashi H, Sassa T, Shibuya T, et al. Effects of sports participation on psychiatric symptoms and brain activations during sports observation in schizophrenia. Translational Psychiatry 2012;2. PMID: 2012160495.

Voruganti LN, Whatham J, Bard E, et al. Going beyond: an adventure- and recreation-based group intervention promotes well-being and weight loss in schizophrenia. Can J Psychiatry. 2006;51(9):575-80. PMID: 17007224.

Vreeland B, Minsky S, Menza M, et al. A program for managing weight gain associated with atypical antipsychotics. Psychiatr Serv. 2003;54(8):1155-7. PMID: 12883145.

Watanabe J, Suzuki Y, Sugai T, et al. The lipid profiles in Japanese patients with schizophrenia treated with antipsychotic agents. Gen Hosp Psychiatry 2012. PMID: 22591814.

Weber M, Wyne K. A cognitive/behavioral group intervention for weight loss in patients treated with atypical antipsychotics. Schizophr Res. 2006;83(1):95-101. PMID: 16507343.

Not a study population of interest

Baptista T, Uzcategui E, Rangel N, et al. Metformin plus sibutramine for olanzapine-associated weight gain and metabolic dysfunction in schizophrenia: a 12-week double-blind, placebo-controlled pilot study. Psychiatry Res. 2008;159(1-2):250-3. PMID: 18374423.

Baptista T, Sandia I, Lacruz A, et al. Insulin counter-regulatory factors, fibrinogen and C-reactive protein during olanzapine administration: effects of the antidiabetic metformin. Int Clin Psychopharmacol. 2007;22(2):69-76. PMID: 17293706.

Baptista T, Rangel N, Fernandez V, et al. Metformin as an adjunctive treatment to control body weight and metabolic dysfunction during olanzapine administration; a multicentric, double-blind, placebo-controlled trial. Schizophr Res. 2007;93(1-3):99-108. PMID: 17490862.

Baptista T, Martinez J, Lacruz A, et al. Metformin for prevention of weight gain and insulin resistance with olanzapine: a double-blind placebo-controlled trial. Can J Psychiatry. 2006;51(3):192-6. PMID: 16618011.

Brown S, Smith E. Can a brief health promotion intervention delivered by mental health key workers improve clients' physical health: A randomized controlled trial. Journal of Mental Health 2009;18(5):372-378.

Deberdt W, Winokur A, Cavazzoni PA, et al. Amantadine for weight gain associated with olanzapine treatment. Eur Neuropsychopharmacol. 2005;15(1):13-21. PMID: 15572269.

Druss DG, von Esenwein SA, Compton MT, et al. A randomized trial of medical care management for community mental health settings: the Primary Care Access, Referral, and Evaluation (PCARE) study. Am J Psychiatry. 2010;167(2):151-9. PMID: 20008945.

Joffe G, Takala P, Tchoukhine E, et al. Orlistat in clozapine- or olanzapine-treated patients with overweight or obesity: a 16-week randomized, double-blind, placebo-controlled trial. J Clin Psychiatry. 2008;69(5):706-11. PMID: 18426261.

Kitabchi AE, Temprosa M, Knowler WC, et al. Role of insulin secretion and sensitivity in the evolution of type 2 diabetes in the diabetes prevention program: effects of lifestyle intervention and metformin. Diabetes. 2005;54(8):2404-14. PMID: 16046308.

Ko YH, Joe SH, Jung IK, et al. Topiramate as an adjuvant treatment with atypical antipsychotics in schizophrenic patients experiencing weight gain. Clin Neuropharmacol. 2005;28(4):169-75. PMID: 16062095.

Methapatara W, Srisurapanont M. Pedometer walking plus motivational interviewing program for Thai schizophrenic patients with obesity or overweight: a 12-week, randomized, controlled trial. Psychiatry Clin Neurosci. 2011;65(4):374-80. PMID: 21682813.

Milano W, Grillo F, Del Mastro A, et al. Appropriate intervention strategies for weight gain induced by olanzapine: a randomized controlled study. Adv Ther. 2007;24(1):123-34. PMID: 17526469.

Tchoukhine E, Takala P, Hakko H, et al. Orlistat in clozapine- or olanzapine-treated patients with overweight or obesity: a 16-week open-label extension phase and both phases of a randomized controlled trial. J Clin Psychiatry. 2011;72(3):326-30. PMID: 20816037.

Young AS, Mintz J and Cohen AN. Using information systems to improve care for persons with schizophrenia. Psychiatr Serv. 2004;55(3):253-5. PMID: 15001724.

Not appropriate setting

Baptista T, Rangel N, El Fakih Y, et al. Rosiglitazone in the assistance of metabolic control during olanzapine administration in schizophrenia: a pilot double-blind, placebo-controlled, 12-week trial. Pharmacopsychiatry. 2009;42(1):14-9. PMID: 19153941.

Cordes J, Th Nker J, Regenbrecht G, et al. Can an early weight management program (WMP) prevent olanzapine (OLZ)-induced disturbances in body weight, blood glucose and lipid metabolism? Twenty-four- and 48-week results from a 6-month randomized trial. World J Biol Psychiatry. 2011; PMID: 21745127.

Covell NH, Weissman EM and Essock SM. Weight gain with clozapine compared to first generation antipsychotic medications. Schizophr Bull. 2004;30(2):229-40. PMID: 15279042.

Del Valle MC, Loebel AD, Murray S, et al. Change in framingham risk score in patients with schizophrenia: a post hoc analysis of a randomized, double-blind, 6-week trial of ziprasidone and olanzapine. Prim Care Companion J Clin Psychiatry. 2006;8(6):329-33. PMID: 17245453.

Lu ML, Lane HY, Lin SK, et al. Adjunctive fluvoxamine inhibits clozapine-related weight gain and metabolic disturbances. J Clin Psychiatry. 2004;65(6):766-71. PMID: 15291653.

Melamed Y, Stein-Reisner O, Gelkopf M, et al. Multi-modal weight control intervention for people with persistent mental disorders. Psychiatr Rehabil J. 2008;31(3):194-200. PMID: 18194946.

Poyurovsky M, Fuchs C, Pashinian A, et al. Attenuating effect of reboxetine on appetite and weight gain in olanzapine-treated schizophrenia patients: a double-blind placebo-controlled study. Psychopharmacology (Berl). 2007;192(3):441-8. PMID: 17310385.

Poyurovsky M, Isaacs I, Fuchs C, et al. Attenuation of olanzapine-induced weight gain with reboxetine in patients with schizophrenia: a double-blind, placebo-controlled study. Am J Psychiatry. 2003;160(2):297-302. PMID: 12562576.

Poyurovsky M, Pashinian A, Gil-Ad I, et al. Olanzapine-induced weight gain in patients with first-episode schizophrenia: a double-blind, placebo-controlled study of fluoxetine addition. Am J Psychiatry. 2002;159(6):1058-60. PMID: 12042201.

Smith RC, Rachakonda S, Dwivedi S, et al. Olanzapine and risperidone effects on appetite and ghrelin in chronic schizophrenic patients. Psychiatry Research 2012.

Wu MK, Wang CK, Bai YM, et al. Outcomes of obese, clozapine-treated inpatients with schizophrenia placed on a six-month diet and physical activity program. Psychiatr Serv. 2007;58(4):544-50. PMID: 17412858.

Wu RR, Zhao JP, Guo XF, et al. Metformin addition attenuates olanzapine-induced weight gain in drug-naive first-episode schizophrenia patients: a double-blind, placebo-controlled study. Am J Psychiatry. 2008;165(3):352-8. PMID: 18245179.

Length of followup less than 2 months

Brown S, Chan K. A randomized controlled trial of a brief health promotion intervention in a population with serious mental illness. J Mental Health. 2006;15(5):543-549.

Ganguli R, Brar JS, Mahmoud R, et al. Assessment of strategies for switching patients from olanzapine to risperidone: a randomized, open-label, rater-blinded study. BMC Med. 2008;6:17. PMID: 18590519.

Kingsbury SJ, Fayek M, Trufasiu D, et al. The apparent effects of ziprasidone on plasma lipids and glucose. J Clin Psychiatry. 2001;62(5):347-9. PMID: 11411816.

No interventions of interest

Afshar H, Roohafza H, Mousavi G, et al. Topiramate add-on treatment in schizophrenia: a randomised, double-blind, placebo-controlled clinical trial. J Psychopharmacol. 2009;23(2):157-62. PMID: 18515465.

Archie S, Wilson JH, Osborne S, et al. Pilot study: access to fitness facility and exercise levels in olanzapine-treated patients. Can J Psychiatry. 2003;48(9):628-32. PMID: 14631884.

Basu R, Thimmaiah TG, Chawla JM, et al. Changes in metabolic syndrome parameters in patients with schizoaffective disorder who participated in a randomized, placebo-controlled trial of topiramate. Asian J Psychiatr. 2009;2(3):106-111.

Bobo WV, Epstein RA, Jr. and Shelton RC. Effects of orally disintegrating vs regular olanzapine tablets on body weight, eating behavior, glycemic and lipid indices, and gastrointestinal hormones: a randomized, open comparison in outpatients with bipolar depression. Ann Clin Psychiatry. 2011;23(3):193-201. PMID: 21808751.

Bowden CL, Calabrese JR, Ketter TA, et al. Impact of lamotrigine and lithium on weight in obese and nonobese patients with bipolar I disorder. Am J Psychiatry. 2006;163(7):1199-201. PMID: 16816224.

Casey DE, Carson WH, Saha AR, et al. Switching patients to aripiprazole from other antipsychotic agents: a multicenter randomized study. Psychopharmacology (Berl). 2003;166(4):391-9. PMID: 12610718.

Emsley R, Turner HJ, Schronen J, et al. Effects of quetiapine and haloperidol on body mass index and glycaemic control: a long-term, randomized, controlled trial. Int J Neuropsychopharmacol. 2005;8(2):175-82. PMID: 15737251.

Essock SM, Schooler NR, Stroup TS, et al. Effectiveness of switching from antipsychotic polypharmacy to monotherapy. Am J Psychiatry. 2011;168(7):702-8. PMID: 21536693.

Goodall E, Oxtoby C, Richards R, et al. A clinical trial of the efficacy and acceptability of {d}-fenfluramine in the treatment of neuroleptic-induced obesity. Br J Psychiatry. 1988;153:208-213.

Henderson DC, Copeland PM, Daley TB, et al. A double-blind, placebo-controlled trial of sibutramine for olanzapine-associated weight gain. Am J Psychiatry. 2005;162(5):954-62. PMID: 15863798.

Henderson DC, Fan X, Copeland PM, et al. A double-blind, placebo-controlled trial of sibutramine for clozapine-associated weight gain. Acta Psychiatr Scand. 2007;115(2):101-5. PMID: 17244173.

Henderson DC, Freudenreich O, Borba CP, et al. Effects of modafinil on weight, glucose and lipid metabolism in clozapine-treated patients with schizophrenia. Schizophr Res. 2011;130(1-3):53-6. PMID: 21565464.

Kemp DE, Calabrese JR, Tran QV, et al. Metabolic syndrome in patients enrolled in a clinical trial of aripiprazole in the maintenance treatment of bipolar I disorder: a post hoc analysis of a randomized, double-blind, placebo-controlled trial. J Clin Psychiatry. 2010;71(9):1138-44. PMID: 20492838.

Kemp DE, Karayal ON, Calabrese JR, et al. Ziprasidone with adjunctive mood stabilizer in the maintenance treatment of bipolar I disorder: Long-term changes in weight and metabolic profiles. Eur Neuropsychopharmacol. 2011. PMID: 21798721.

Kinon BJ, Basson BR, Gilmore JA, et al. Strategies for switching from conventional antipsychotic drugs or risperidone to olanzapine. J Clin Psychiatry. 2000;61(11):833-40. PMID: 11105736.

Kinon BJ, Chen L, Ascher-Svanum H, et al. Early response to antipsychotic drug therapy as a clinical marker of subsequent response in the treatment of schizophrenia. Neuropsychopharmacology. 2010;35(2):581-90. PMID: 19890258.

Kinon BJ, Liu-Seifert H, Ahl J, et al. Longitudinal effect of olanzapine on fasting serum lipids: a randomized, prospective, 4-month study. Ann N Y Acad Sci. 2004;1032:295-6. PMID: 15677433.

Kinon BJ, Volavka J, Stauffer V, et al. Standard and higher dose of olanzapine in patients with schizophrenia or schizoaffective disorder: a randomized, double-blind, fixed-dose study. J Clin Psychopharmacol. 2008;28(4):392-400. PMID: 18626265.

Kolotkin RL, Corey-Lisle PK, Crosby RD, et al. Changes in weight and weight-related quality of life in a multicentre, randomized trial of aripiprazole versus standard of care. Eur Psychiatry. 2008;23(8):561-6. PMID: 18374544.

Kusumi I, Honda M, Uemura K, et al. Effect of olanzapine orally disintegrating tablet versus oral standard tablet on body weight in patients with schizophrenia: a randomized open-label trial. Prog Neuropsychopharmacol Biol Psychiatry. 2011;:. PMID: 22119746.

McCreadie RG, Kelly C, Connolly M, et al. Dietary improvement in people with schizophrenia: randomised controlled trial. Br J Psychiatry. 2005;187:346-51. PMID: 16199794.

McElroy SL, Frye MA, Altshuler LL, et al. A 24-week, randomized, controlled trial of adjunctive sibutramine versus topiramate in the treatment of weight gain in overweight or obese patients with bipolar disorders. Bipolar Disord. 2007;9(4):426-34. PMID: 17547588.

McIntyre RS, Mancini DA, McCann S, et al. Topiramate versus bupropion SR when added to mood stabilizer therapy for the depressive phase of bipolar disorder: a preliminary single-blind study. Bipolar Disord. 2002;4(3):207-13. PMID: 12180276.

McIntyre RS, McElroy SL, Eudicone JM, et al. A 52-week, double-blind evaluation of the metabolic effects of aripiprazole and lithium in bipolar I disorder. Primary Care Companion to the Journal of Clinical Psychiatry 2011;13(6). PMID: 2012045221.

McQuade RD, Stock E, Marcus R, et al. A comparison of weight change during treatment with olanzapine or aripiprazole: results from a randomized, double-blind study. J Clin Psychiatry. 2004;65 Suppl 18:47-56. PMID: 15600384.

Meltzer HY, Bonaccorso S, Bobo WV, et al. A 12-month randomized, open-label study of the metabolic effects of olanzapine and risperidone in psychotic patients: Influence of valproic acid augmentation. Journal of Clinical Psychiatry 2011;72(12):1602-1610. PMID: 2012003061.

Newcomer JW, Meyer JM, Baker RA, et al. Changes in non-high-density lipoprotein cholesterol levels and triglyceride/high-density lipoprotein cholesterol ratios among patients randomized to aripiprazole versus olanzapine. Schizophr Res. 2008;106(2-3):300-7. PMID: 18973991.

Rosenheck RA, Davis S, Covell N, et al. Does switching to a new antipsychotic improve outcomes? Data from the CATIE Trial. Schizophr Res. 2009;107(1):22-9. PMID: 18993031.

Roy Chengappa K, Kupfer DJ, Parepally H, et al. A placebo-controlled, random-assignment, parallel-group pilot study of adjunctive topiramate for patients with schizoaffective disorder, bipolar type. Bipolar Disord. 2007;9(6):609-17. PMID: 17845276.

Roy Chengappa KN, Schwarzman LK, Hulihan JF, et al. Adjunctive topiramate therapy in patients receiving a mood stabilizer for bipolar I disorder: a randomized, placebo-controlled trial. J Clin Psychiatry. 2006;67(11):1698-706. PMID: 17196048.

Schreiner A, Niehaus D, Shuriquie NA, et al. Metabolic Effects of Paliperidone Extended Release Versus Oral Olanzapine in Patients With Schizophrenia: A Prospective, Randomized, Controlled Trial. J Clin Psychopharmacol 2012;32(4):449-457. PMID: 22722501.

Xiang YT, Wang CY, Ungvari GS, et al. Weight changes and their associations with demographic and clinical characteristics in risperidone maintenance treatment for schizophrenia. Pharmacopsychiatry. 2011;44(4):135-41. PMID: 21710403.

No outcomes of interest

Acil AA, Dogan S, Dogan O. The effects of physical exercises to mental state and quality of life in patients with schizophrenia. J Psychiatr Ment Health Nurs. 2008;15(10):808-15. PMID: 19012672.

Chafetz L, White M, Collins-Bride G, et al. Clinical trial of wellness training: health promotion for severely mentally ill adults. J Nerv Ment Dis. 2008;196(6):475-83. PMID: 18552625.

Goodrich DE, Kilbourne AM, Lai Z, et al. Design and rationale of a randomized controlled trial to reduce cardiovascular disease risk for patients with bipolar disorder. Contemp Clin Trials 2012;33(4):666-78. PMID: 22386799.

Jerome GJ, Dalcin AT, Young DR, et al. Rationale, design and baseline data for the Activating Consumers to Exercise through Peer Support (ACE trial): A randomized controlled trial to increase fitness among adults with mental illness. Mental Health and Physical Activity 2012.

Kilbourne AM, Post EP, Nossek A, et al. Improving medical and psychiatric outcomes among individuals with bipolar disorder: a randomized controlled trial. Psychiatr Serv. 2008;59(7):760-8. PMID: 18586993.

Kim SW, Chung YC, Lee YH, et al. Paliperidone ER versus risperidone for neurocognitive function in patients with schizophrenia: a randomized, open-label, controlled trial. Int Clin Psychopharmacol 2012. PMID: 22809972.

Muscatello MR, Bruno A, Pandolfo G, et al. Topiramate augmentation of clozapine in schizophrenia: a double-blind, placebo-controlled study. J Psychopharmacol. 2011;25(5):667-74. PMID: 20615930.

Scheewe TW, Takken T, Kahn RS, et al. Effects of Exercise Therapy on Cardiorespiratory Fitness in Schizophrenia Patients. Med Sci Sports Exerc 2012. PMID: 22525773

Appendix F. Study Characteristics Table

Table F-1. Study characteristics table for SMI comparative effectiveness review[a]

Study Country Randomized Patients (N)	Patient Characteristics	Intervention	Comparator	Outcomes Timing	Effectiveness Rating Funding	Study Quality: Hard Outcomes Soft Outcomes
Alvarez-Jimenez, 2006[1] Europe 61	Mean age: 26.8 Female N: 15 Male N: 46 Nonwhite: NR Schizophrenia N: 61 Bipolar N: NR Other N: NR	Early behavioral intervention: 10–14 weekly or twice weekly individual therapy sessions following a flexible but manualized program, provided by a master's-level psychologist, focused on education, motivation, and skills training to enhance control over factors associated with antipsychotic weight gain.	Enhanced usual care "designed to provide patients with the same physical care that is offered in a comprehensive early psychosis program."	BMI Weight (kg) 3 months, 4 months, 6 months, 12 months, 24 months	Mixed (4) Marques de Valddecilla Public Foundation– government	Good NA
Assuncao, 2006[2] South America 54	Mean age: 35.2 Female N: 22 Male N: 32 Nonwhite: 18 Schizophrenia N: 54 Bipolar N: 0 Other N: 0	Nizatidine 600 mg/day All participants were continued on their pretrial dose of olanzapine (5-20 mg/day).	Placebo All participants were continued on their pretrial dose of olanzapine (5-20 mg/day).	Weight (kg) Total Cholesterol (mg/dl) LDL (mg/dl) Discontinuation due to adverse event "Treatment emergent adverse event" Psychiatric Symptom Severity: EPRS 4 weeks, 8 weeks, 12 weeks	Efficacy (2) Industry	Good Good

F-1

Study Country Randomized Patients (N)	Patient Characteristics	Intervention	Comparator	Outcomes Timing	Effectiveness Rating Funding	Study Quality: Hard Outcomes Soft Outcomes
Atmaca, 2003[3] Europe 35	Mean age: 27.9 Female N: 14 Male N: 21 Nonwhite: NR Schizophrenia N: 35 Bipolar N: N:NR Other N: NR	Nizatidine 300 mg/day All participants were continued on their pretrial dose of olanzapine.	Placebo All participants were continued on their pretrial dose of olanzapine.	BMI Weight (kg) Psychiatric Symptom Severity: PANSS Any adverse event 8 weeks	Efficacy (0) Not reported or unclear	Fair Fair
Atmaca, 2004[4] Europe 28	Mean age: 30.2 Female N: 12 Male N: 13 The sex of the 3 participants who did not complete the study was not reported. Nonwhite: NR Schizophrenia N: 28 Bipolar N: NR Other N: NR	Quetiapine 300 - 750 mg/day (mean dose 479 mg/day) + nizatidine 300 mg/day	Quetiapine 300 - 750 mg/day (mean dose 493 mg/day) + placebo	BMI Weight (kg) Psychiatric Symptom Severity: PANSS Leptin levels 2 months	Efficacy (0) Not reported or unclear	Fair Fair
Ball, 2011[5] US 36	Mean age: 47.0 Female N: 11 Male N: 25 Nonwhite: 11 Schizophrenia N: 36 Bipolar N: NR Other N: NR	Atomoxetine 120 mg/day All participants attended weekly group counseling, exercise sessions 3 times per week, and 10 weeks of Weight Watchers. All participants were continued on their pretrial dose of clozapine or olanzapine.	Placebo All participants attended weekly group counseling, exercise sessions 3 times per week, and 10 weeks of Weight Watchers. All participants were continued on their pretrial dose of clozapine or olanzapine.	Weight (kg) LDL (mg/dl) 9 weeks, 24 weeks, 6 months	Mixed (4) Government, Industry	Fair Fair

F-2

Study Country Randomized Patients (N)	Patient Characteristics	Intervention	Comparator	Outcomes Timing	Effectiveness Rating Funding	Study Quality: Hard Outcomes Soft Outcomes
Borba, 2011[6] US 20	Mean age: 51.1 Female N: 7 Male N: 13 Nonwhite: 2 Schizophrenia N: 20 Bipolar N: NR Other N: NR	Ramelteon 8 mg/day All participants were continued on their pretrial medications.	Placebo All participants were continued on their pretrial medications.	BMI Weight (kg) HbA1c (%) Total cholesterol (mg/dl) LDL (mg/dl) 2 months	Efficacy (0) Government, Industry	Fair NA
Brar, 2005[7] US 71	Mean age: 40.3 Female N: 42 Male N: 29 Nonwhite: 36 Schizophrenia N: 71 Bipolar N: 0 Other N: 0	20 manualized behavioral therapy sessions, twice weekly for 6 weeks followed by weekly for 8 weeks, covering diet, nutrition, exercise, and self-monitoring of behavioral changes.	Usual care	BMI Weight (kg) Systolic blood pressure (mmHg) Diastolic blood pressure (mmHg) 14 weeks	Efficacy (1) Industry	Fair Fair
Brown, 2011[8] US 89	Mean age: 44.6 Female N: 54 Male N: 35 Nonwhite: 35 Schizophrenia N: NR Bipolar N: NR Other N: NR	Recovering Energy Through Nutrition and Exercise for Weight Loss (RENEW): weekly individual visits for 12 weeks followed by monthly individual visits and weekly phone calls for the following 3 months. Sessions focused on weight loss strategies including social support, goal setting, skills training, and compensatory strategies for cognitive impairments.	Usual care	Weight (lb) 3 months, 6 months	Efficacy (1) Government, Industry	Fair Fair

Study Country Randomized Patients (N)	Patient Characteristics	Intervention	Comparator	Outcomes Timing	Effectiveness Rating Funding	Study Quality: Hard Outcomes Soft Outcomes
Bustillo, 2003[9] US 30	Mean age: 34.5 Female N: 6 Male N: 24 Nonwhite: 15 Schizophrenia N: 30 Bipolar N: NR Other N: NR	Olanzapine 10 mg/day plus fluoxetine 20–60 mg/day (mean dose 56 mg/day)	Olanzapine 10 mg/day plus placebo	Weight (kg) Psychiatric Symptom Severity: PANSS-Positive Symptoms Psychiatric Symptom Severity: HAM-D Adverse Event: Extrapyramidal symptoms 4 months	Efficacy (2) Government, Industry	Fair Fair
Carrizo, 2009[10] South America 61	Mean age: 38.9 Female N: NR Male N: NR Nonwhite: 50 Schizophrenia N: 52 Bipolar N: 2 The numbers for diagnoses are based on the number of individuals who completed the trial, which was 54. 61 were randomized Other N: NR	Metformin 500–1000 mg/day All participants continued taking their pretrial clozapine, although it was unclear if dosing was changed during the trial. Mean starting dose of clozapine for intervention arm was 180 mg/day.	Placebo All participants continued taking their pretrial clozapine, although it was unclear if dosing was changed during the trial. Mean starting dose of clozapine for placebo arm was 207 mg/day.	BMI Weight (kg) HbA1c (%) Systolic blood pressure (mmHg) Diastolic blood pressure (mmHg) Psychiatric Symptom Severity: BPRS 7 weeks, 14 weeks	Efficacy (1) Government, Industry	Fair Fair

Study / Country / Randomized Patients (N)	Patient Characteristics	Intervention	Comparator	Outcomes / Timing	Effectiveness Rating / Funding	Study Quality: Hard Outcomes / Soft Outcomes
Cavazzoni, 2003[11] US 175	Mean age: NR Female N: NR Male N: NR Nonwhite: NR Schizophrenia N: 169 Bipolar N:NR Other N: NR 175 randomized, 169 completed and analyzed.	This was a 3-arm trial with 2 active arms. Arm 1: Pretrial dose of olanzapine plus nizatidine 300 mg/day Arm 2: Pretrial dose of olanzapine plus nizatidine 600 mg/day	Pretrial dose of olanzapine + placebo	Weight (b) Psychiatic Symptom Severity: BPRS 1, 2, 3, 4, 5, 6, 8, 12, and 16 weeks	Efficacy (1) Industry	Fair Poor
Deberdt, 2008[12] US 133	Mean age: 44.0 Female N: NR Male N: NR Nonwhite: NR Schizophrenia N: 133 Bipolar N: 0 Other N: 0	Antipsychotic switching: FROM olanzapine 10-20 mg/day TO quetiapine 300-800 mg/day	CONTINUE olanzapine 10-20 mg/day Comparators were continued on olanzapine although the dose of olanzapine could be changed during the trial.	BMI Weight (kg) HbA1c (%) Total cholesterol (mmol/L) LDL (mmol/L) 1, 2, 3, 5, 7, 10, 12, 16, 18, 22, and 24 weeks	Mixed (5) Industry	Fair Fair
Elmslie, 2006[13] Australia/New Zealand 60	Mean age: 42.0 Female N: 49 Male N: 11 Nonwhite: NR Schizophrenia N: NR Bipolar N:60 Other N: NR	Carnitine L-tartrate 15 mg/kg/day	Placebo control	BMI Weight (kg) Waist circumference change (cm) 26 weeks	Mixed (3) Private foundation	Good Good

Study Country Randomized Patients (N)	Patient Characteristics	Intervention	Comparator	Outcomes Timing	Effectiveness Rating Funding	Study Quality: Hard Outcomes Soft Outcomes
Evans, 2005[14] Australia/New Zealand 51	Mean age: 34.2 Female N: 29 Male N: 22 Nonwhite: NR Schizophrenia N: 38 Bipolar N: 8 Other N: 5	Nutrition education: 6 planned, 1 hour contacts including education on diet, nutrition, physical activity, and exercise and assistance in goal setting, provided every 2 weeks by an accredited practicing dietitian.	Usual care	BMI Weight (kg) 3 months, 6 months	Efficacy (1) Industry	Poor Poor
Fleischhacker, 2010[15] Europe, Africa 207	Mean age: 39.0 Female N: 73 Male N: 134 Nonwhite: 10 Schizophrenia N: 207 Bipolar N: 0 Other N: 0	Aripiprazole 5–15 mg/day; mean dose = 11.1 mg/day All participants were continued on their prestudy dose of clozapine throughout the trial.	Placebo All participants were continued on their prestudy dose of clozapine throughout the trial.	BMI Weight (kg) Total Cholesterol (mg/dl) LDL (mg/dl) Discontinuation due to adverse event All-cause mortality HRQOL/Physical function: Subjective Well Being Under Neuroleptics Scale score 2, 4, 6, 8, 10, 12, 14, and 16 weeks	Mixed (3) Industry	Good Good
Forsberg, 2008[16] Europe 41	Mean age: 41.0 Female N: 16 Male N: 25 Nonwhite: NR Schizophrenia N: NR Bipolar N: NR Other N: NR	Multimodal lifestyle intervention of 70 group visits over 12 months, with activities including fitness exercises, practice buying and preparing food, learning to monitor heart rate, and activity scheduling. Participants received 50% subsidy on entrance and rental fees at sports centers.	Once weekly art class for 12 months.	BMI Weight (kg) HbA1c (%) Systolic blood pressure (mm Hg) Diastolic blood pressure (mm Hg) Smoking cessation Number of participants meeting criteria for Metabolic syndrome 13.5 months	Mixed (4) Government, Private foundation	Fair NA

Study / Country / Randomized Patients (N)	Patient Characteristics	Intervention	Comparator	Outcomes / Timing	Effectiveness Rating / Funding	Study Quality: Hard Outcomes / Soft Outcomes
Gillhoff, 2010[17] Europe 50	Mean age: 48.0 Female N: 23 Male N: 27 Nonwhite: NR Schizophrenia N: NR Bipolar N: 50 Other N: NR	Multimodal lifestyle intervention including weekly fitness training, 7 psychotherapeutic/educational sessions, and 4 cooking and nutrition classes over the course of 5 months.	Wait list / Usual Care	BMI Weight (kg) HbA1c (%) Total cholesterol (mmol/L) LDL (mmol/L) Systolic blood pressure (mm Hg) Diastolic blood pressure (mm Hg) 5 months, 11 months	Efficacy (2) Industry	Fair NA
Graham, 2005[18] US 21	Mean age: NR Female N: 9 Male N: 12 Nonwhite: 5 Schizophrenia N: 18 Bipolar N: 3 Other N: 0	Amantadine up to 300 mg/day (no further dosing details given) + 12 weekly sessions of healthy lifestyle education program and 3 month membership to gym or commercial weight loss program	Placebo + 12 sessions of healthy lifestyle education program and 3 month membership to gym or commercial weight loss program	BMI Weight (lb) 1 month, 2 months, 3 months	Mixed (3) Government, Industry	Poor NA
Hoffmann, 2012[19] US, Europe, Asia, Middle East, Mexico 199	Mean age: 38.5 Female N: 79 Male N: 120 Nonwhite: 112 Schizophrenia N: 199 Bipolar N: NR Other N: NR	This was a 3-arm trial with 2 active arms. Arm 1: Pretrial dose of olanzapine plus metformin 1000-1500 mg/day, followed by amantadine 200 mg/day if metformin was ineffective Arm 2: Pretrial dose of olanzapine plus amantadine 200 mg/day, followed by metformin 1000-1500 mg/day if amantadine was ineffective	Pretrial dose of olanzapine only	BMI Weight (kg) HgA1c (%) Total cholesterol (mmol/L) LDL (mmol/L) Discontinuation due to adverse event Psychiatric Symptom Severity: EPRS Psychiatric Symptom Severity: CGI Psychiatric Symptom Severity: MADRS 22 weeks	Mixed (3) Industry	Poor Poor

F-7

Study Country Randomized Patients (N)	Patient Characteristics	Intervention	Comparator	Outcomes Timing	Effectiveness Rating Funding	Study Quality: Hard Outcomes Soft Outcomes
Karagianis, 2009[20] US, Canada, Europe, Mexico 149	Mean age: 39.0 Female N: 68 Male N: 81 Nonwhite: 71 Schizophrenia N: 106 Bipolar N: 41 Other N: 2	Antipsychotic-switching: FROM standard tablets of olanzapine 5-20 mg/day TO orally disintegrating olanzapine 5-20 mg/day (mean dose 14.3 mg/day)	CONTINUE standard tablets of olanzapine 5-20 mg/day (mean dose 14.9 mg/day)	BMI Weight (kg) HbA1c (%) Total cholesterol (mg/dl) LDL (mg/dl) Systolic blood pressure (mm Hg) Diastolic blood pressure (mm Hg) Discontinuation due to adverse event HRQOL/Physical Function: Subjective Well Being Under Neuroleptics Scale score 2, 4, 6, 8, 10, 12, 14, and 16 weeks	Mixed (4) Industry	Good Good
Khazaal, 2007[21] Europe 61	Mean age: 40.7 Female N: 33 Male N: 28 Nonwhite: NR Schizophrenia N: 49 Bipolar N: 5 Other N: 7	12 weekly CBT-based manualized groups, provided by a master's-level psychologist, covering nutrition, diet, activity, exercise, and psychoeducation	One 2-hour nutrition education group	BMI Weight (kg) 3 months, 6 months	Efficacy (1) Not reported or unclear	Fair NA

Study / Country / Randomized Patients (N)	Patient Characteristics	Intervention	Comparator	Outcomes / Timing	Effectiveness Rating / Funding	Study Quality: Hard Outcomes / Soft Outcomes
Kwon, 2006[22] Asia 48	Mean age: 31.3 Female N: 33 Male N: 15 Nonwhite: NR Schizophrenia N: 48 Bipolar N: 0 Other N: 0	8 session CBT weight management program focused on diet and exercise management, with a dietician and an exercise coordinator. All participants continued their pretrial dose of olanzapine (5-20 mg/day).	Usual care All participants continued their pretrial dose of olanzapine (5-20 mg/day).	BMI Weight (kg) Systolic blood pressure (mm Hg) Diastolic blood pressure (mm Hg) HRQOL/Physical Function: WHO-QOL-BREF, physical health subscore 4 weeks, 8 weeks, 12 weeks	Efficacy (1) Industry	Fair Poor
Littrell, 2003[23] US 70	Mean age: 34.1 Female N: 27 Male N: 43 Nonwhite: 18 Schizophrenia N: 70 Bipolar N: 0 Other N: 0	Olanzapine plus 16-session manualized education intervention administered by a master's-level clinician, focused on diet, nutrition, exercise, goal and activity setting, and self-monitoring.	Olanzapine only	BMI Weight (lb) 4 months, 6 months	Mixed (3) Industry	Good NA
Mauri, 2008[24] Europe 49	Mean age: 38.9 Female N: 28 Male N: 21 Nonwhite: NR Schizophrenia N: 5 Bipolar N: 43 Other N: 1	5–7 psychoeducational groups on diet, exercise, nutrition, self-monitoring, and goal-setting. All participants were continued on their pretrial dose of olanzapine.	Usual care All participants were continued on their pretrial dose of olanzapine.	BMI Weight (kg) Total Cholesterol (mg/dl) LDL (mg/d) Psychiatric Symptom Severity: GAF Adverse Event: drug-related 3 months	Efficacy (1) Industry	Poor Poor

| Study | Patient Characteristics | Intervention | Comparator | Outcomes | Effectiveness Rating | Study Quality: Hard Outcomes |
| Country | | | | | | |
Randomized Patients (N)				Timing	Funding	Soft Outcomes
McDonnell, 2011[25] "26 countries worldwide" – no further details provided 1065	Mean age: 38.9 Female N: 459 Male N: 856 The sex of the participants starting the trial was reported; the total participants starting n=1315, but this lead-in period was not randomized. By the point of the randomized part of the trial, there were 1065 individuals, but the breakdown for sex was not reported. Nonwhite: 299 Schizophrenia N: 921 Bipolar N: NR Other N: NR	Antipsychotic switching: FROM oral tablets of olanzapine TO long-acting injectable olanzapine 45 mg every 4 weeks	Continue oral tablets of olanzapine 10-20 mg/day (mean dose 14.3 mg/day)	BMI Weight (kg) Total Cholesterol (mg/dl) LDL (mg/dl) Discontinuation due to adverse event Adverse event: "Treatment-emergent adverse event" 24 weeks	Efficacy (2) Industry	Fair Fair
McElroy, 2012[26] US 42	Mean age: 33.7 Female N: 13 Male N: 29 Nonwhite: 9 Schizophrenia N: 1 Bipolar N: 42 Other N: NR	Zonisamide 100-600 mg/day (mean dose 380 mg/day) All participants were registered to receive Personal Wellness Solution Counseling. All participants continued their pretrial dose of olanzapine.	Placebo All participants were registered to receive Personal Wellness Solution Counseling. All participants continued their pretrial dose of olanzapine.	BMI Weight (kg) Total cholesterol (mg/dl) LDL (mg/dl) Systolic blood pressure (mm Hg) Diastolic blood pressure (mm Hg) Psychiatric Symptom Severity: CGI-S, bipolar version 1, 2, 3, 4, 6, 8, 10, 12, 14, and 16 weeks	Efficacy (2) Industry	Good Good

Study Country Randomized Patients (N)	Patient Characteristics	Intervention	Comparator	Outcomes Timing	Effectiveness Rating Funding	Study Quality: Hard Outcomes Soft Outcomes
McKibbin, 2006[27] US 64	Mean age: 54.0 Female N: 20 Male N: 37 Nonwhite: 22 Schizophrenia N: 57 Bipolar N: NR Other N: NR 64 randomized, 52 completed and analyzed	Diabetes Awareness and Rehabilitation Training (DART): 90 minute, weekly, manualized sessions (up to 24 sessions, mean number of sessions 16.2), based on Social Cognitive Theory, addressing diabetes, nutrition, lifestyle, exercise, self-empowerment, self-monitoring, and ncentives	Usual care plus 3 brochures from the American Diabetes Association on diabetes management	BMI HbA1c (%) LDL (mg/d) Systolic blood pressure (mm Hg) Diastolic blood pressure (mm Hg) 6 months, 12 months	Efficacy (2) Government	Fair Fair
Narula, 2010[28] Asia 72	Mean age: 31.1 Female N: 23 Male N: 44 Nonwhite: NR Schizophrenia N: 67 Bipolar N: NR Other N: NR 72 randomized, 67 completed and analyzed.	Olanzapine 5-2C mg/day + topiramate 100 mg/day	Olanzapine 5-20 mg/day + placebo	BMI Weight (kg) Total cholesterol (mg/dl) LDL (mg/d) Systolic blood pressure (mm Hg) Diastolic blood pressure (mm Hg) Psychiatric Symptom Severity: PANSS 3 months	Efficacy (1) Not reported or unclear	Fair Fair
Newcomer, 2008[29] "Multinational" 173	Mean age: 39.2 Female N: 62 Male N: 111 Nonwhite: 55 Schizophrenia N: 173 Bipolar N: NR Other N: NR	Antipsychotic switching: FROM olanzapine at 10-20 mg/day (mean 15.9 mg/day) TO aripiprazole 15 mg/day (mean 16.0 mg/day)	CONTINUE olanzapine at 10-20 mg/day (mean 15.9 mg/day)	Weight (kg) Total Cholesterol (mg/dl) LDL (mg/d) Any Adverse Event Psychiatric Symptom Severity: CGI-I 6 weeks, 8 weeks, 12 weeks, 14 weeks	Mixed (4) Industry	Fair Fair

Study Country Randomized Patients (N)	Patient Characteristics	Intervention	Comparator	Outcomes Timing	Effectiveness Rating Funding	Study Quality: Hard Outcomes Soft Outcomes
Nickel, 2005[30] Europe 49	Mean age: 34.9 Female N: 49 Male N: 0 Nonwhite: NR Schizophrenia N: 20 Bipolar N: NR Other N: NR	Topiramate 250 mg/day	Placebo	Weight (kg) HRQOL/Physical Function: SF36-Physical Functioning HRQOL/Physical Function: SF36-Role 10 weeks	Efficacy (1) Not reported or unclear	Fair Fair
Skrinar, 2005[31] US 30	Mean age: 37.8 Female N: 20 Male N: 10 Nonwhite: NR Schizophrenia N: NR Bipolar N: NR Other N: NR	48 exercise sessions (4 per week) plus 12 health education sessions (1 per week), including healthy eating, weight management, adequate amounts of exercise, stress relief, spirituality and wellness, and individual planning to incorporate wellness activities. Participants attended an average of 31 exercise sessions.	Usual care	BMI Weight (kg) Total cholesterol (mg/dl) Psychiatric Symptom Severity: SCL-90, SF-36, QOL 3 months	Efficacy (2) Industry	Fair Fair

Study Country Randomized Patients (N)	Patient Characteristics	Intervention	Comparator	Outcomes Timing	Effectiveness Rating Funding	Study Quality: Hard Outcomes Soft Outcomes
Stroup, 2011[32] US 215	Mean age: 41.0 Female N: 78 Male N: 137 Nonwhite: 92 Schizophrenia N: 215 Bipolar N: NR Other N: NR	Antipsychotic switching: FROM olanzapine at 5-20 mg/day (mean 18.5 mg/day) OR quetiapine at 200-~200 mg/day (mean 502 mg/day) OR risperidone 1-16 mg/day (mean 4.1 mg/day) TO aripiprazole 5-30 mg/day (mean 16.9 mg/day) PLUS a manualized behavioral intervention occurring weekly for 4 weeks and monthly thereafter, including diet, exercise, and education on reducing risk of cardiovascular disease.	CONTINUE: olanzapine 5-20 mg/day (mean 18.0 mg/day) OR quetiapine 200-1200 mg/day (mean 572 mg/day) OR risperidone 1-16 mg/day (mean 4.1 mg/day). Doses of medication could be adjusted during the trial, but medication could not be switched. PLUS a manualized behavioral intervention occurring weekly for 4 weeks and monthly thereafter, including diet, exercise, and education on reducing risk of cardiovascular disease.	BMI Weight (kg) HbA1c (%) Total cholesterol (mg/dl) LDL (mg/dl) Other CVD Summary Risk Score Discontinuation due to adverse event Adverse Event: Death Adverse Event: Hospitalization Adverse Event: Any serious adverse event Psychiatric Symptom Severity: CGI 24 weeks	Mixed (5) Government, Industry	Good Good
Wang, 2012[33] Asia 72	Mean age: NR Female N: 32 Male N: 34 Nonwhite: NR Schizophrenia N: 66 Bipolar N: 0 Other N: 0	Metformin 1000 mg/day (250 mg bid for first 3 days; 500 mg bid for remainder)	Placebo	Discontinuation due to adverse event BMI Weight (kg) Fasting glucose 4 weeks, 8 weeks, 12 weeks	Efficacy (2) Scientific Research Fund of Liaoning Science and Technology Agency, China	Fair Fair

Study Country Randomized Patients (N)	Patient Characteristics	Intervention	Comparator	Outcomes Timing	Effectiveness Rating Funding	Study Quality: Hard Outcomes	Soft Outcomes
Wu, 2008[34] Asia 128	Mean age: 26.3 Female N: 64 Male N: 64 Nonwhite: NR Schizophrenia N: 128 Bipolar N: 0 Other N: 0	This was a 4-arm trial with 3 active arms. Arm 1: Metformin 750 mg/day Arm 2: Manualized lifestyle intervention including sessions on diet, exercise, medication adherence, goal setting, and activity scheduling. Some sessions included family; some sessions were provided by an exercise physiologist or a dietician. Arm 3: Metformin 750 mg/day and manualized lifestyle intervention	Usual care plus placebo	BMI Weight (kg) Discontinuation due to adverse event Insulin level (µIU/mL) Psychiatric Symptom Severity: PANSS 4 weeks, 8 weeks, 12 weeks	Mixed (5) Government	Good	Good
Wu, 2012[35] Asia 84	Mean age: NR Female N: 84 Male N: 0 Nonwhite: 84 Schizophrenia N: 84 Bipolar N: 0 Other N: 0	Metformin 1000 mg/day	Placebo	BMI Weight (kg) Discontinuation due to adverse event Fasting blood glucose in mmol/L 1,2,3,4,5,6 months	Mixed (3) Government	Good	Good

[a]Data for major outcomes are available from the authors upon request.
Abbreviations: BMI=body mass index; BPRS=Brief Psychiatric Rating Scale; CBT=cognitive behavioral training; CGI=clinical global impression; CVD=cardiovascular disease; GAF=global assessment of functioning; HAM-D=Hamilton Depression Rating Scale; HbA1c=glycosylated hemoglobin; HRQOL=health-related quality of life; LDL=low-density lipoprotein; MADRS=Montgomery-Asberg Depression Rating Scale; NA=not applicable; NR=not reported; PANSS=positive and negative syndrome scale; WHO-QOL-BREF=World Health Organization-Quality of Life (abbreviated)

References Cited in Appendix F

1. 1. Alvarez-Jimenez M, Gonzalez-Blanch C, Vazquez-Barquero JL, et al. Attenuation of antipsychotic-induced weight gain with early behavioral intervention in drug-naive first-episode psychosis patients: A randomized controlled trial. J Clin Psychiatry. 2006;67(8):1253-60. PMID: 16965204.

2. Assuncao SS, Ruschel SI, Rosa Lde C, et al. Weight gain management in patients with schizophrenia during treatment with olanzapine in association with nizatidine. Rev Bras Psiquiatr. 2006;28(4):270-6. PMID: 17242805.

3. Atmaca M, Kuloglu M, Tezcan E, et al. Nizatidine treatment and its relationship with leptin levels in patients with olanzapine-induced weight gain. Hum Psychopharmacol. 2003;18(6):457-61. PMID: 12923824.

4. Atmaca M, Kuloglu M, Tezcan E, et al. Nizatidine for the treatment of patients with quetiapine-induced weight gain. Hum Psychopharmacol. 2004;19(1):37-40. PMID: 14716710.

5. Ball MP, Warren KR, Feldman S, et al. Placebo-controlled trial of atomoxetine for weight reduction in people with schizophrenia treated with clozapine or olanzapine. Clin Schizophr Relat Psychoses. 2011;5(1):17-25. PMID; 21459735.

6. Borba CP, Fan X, Copeland PM, et al. Placebo-controlled pilot study of ramelteon for adiposity and lipids in patients with schizophrenia. J Clin Psychopharmacol. 2011;31(5):653-8. PMID: 21869685.

7. Brar JS, Ganguli R, Pandina G, et al. Effects of behavioral therapy on weight loss in overweight and obese patients with schizophrenia or schizoaffective disorder. J Clin Psychiatry. 2005;66(2):205-12. PMID: 15705006.

8. Brown C, Goetz J, Hamera E. Weight loss intervention for people with serious mental illness: a randomized controlled trial of the RENEW program. Psychiatr Serv. 2011;62(7):800-2. PMID: 21724796.

9. Bustillo JR, Lauriello J, Parker K, et al. Treatment of weight gain with fluoxetine in olanzapine-treated schizophrenic outpatients. Neuropsychopharmacology. 2003;28(3):527-9. PMID: 12629532.

10. Carrizo E, Fernandez V, Connell L, et al. Extended release metformin for metabolic control assistance during prolonged clozapine administration: a 14 week, double-blind, parallel group, placebo-controlled study. Schizophr Res. 2009;113(1):19-26. PMID: 19515536.

11. Cavazzoni P, Tanaka Y, Roychowdhury SM, et al. Nizatidine for prevention of weight gain with olanzapine: a double-blind placebo-controlled trial. Eur Neuropsychopharmacol. 2003;13(2):81-5. PMID: 12650950.

12. Deberdt W, Lipkovich I, Heinloth AN, et al. Double-blind, randomized trial comparing efficacy and safety of continuing olanzapine versus switching to quetiapine in overweight or obese patients with schizophrenia or schizoaffective disorder. Ther Clin Risk Manag. 2008;4(4):713-20. PMID: 19209252.

13. Elmslie JL, Porter RJ, Joyce PR, et al. Carnitine does not improve weight loss outcomes in valproate-treated bipolar patients consuming an energy-restricted, low-fat diet. Bipolar Disord. 2006;8(5 Pt 1):503-7. PMID: 17042889.

14. Evans S, Newton R, Higgins S. Nutritional intervention to prevent weight gain in patients commenced on olanzapine: a randomized controlled trial. Aust N Z J Psychiatry. 2005;39(6):479-86. PMID: 15943650.

15. Fleischhacker WW, Heikkinen ME, Olie JP, et al. Effects of adjunctive treatment with aripiprazole on body weight and clinical efficacy in schizophrenia patients treated with clozapine: a randomized, double-blind, placebo-controlled trial. Int J Neuropsychopharmacol. 2010;13(8):1115-25. PMID: 20459883.

16. Forsberg KA, Bjorkman T, Sandman PO, et al. Physical health--a cluster randomized controlled lifestyle intervention among persons with a psychiatric disability and their staff. Nord J Psychiatry. 2008;62(6):486-95. PMID: 18843564.

17. Gillhoff K, Gaab J, Emini L, et al. Effects of a multimodal lifestyle intervention on body mass index in patients with bipolar disorder: a

randomized controlled trial. Prim Care Companion J Clin Psychiatry. 2010;12(5). PMID: 21274359.

18. Graham KA, Gu H, Lieberman JA, et al. Double-blind, placebo-controlled investigation of amantadine for weight loss in subjects who gained weight with olanzapine. Am J Psychiatry. 2005;162(9):1744-6. PMID: 16135638.

19. Hoffmann VP, Case M, Jacobson JG. Assessment of treatment algorithms including amantadine, metformin, and zonisamide for the prevention of weight gain with olanzapine: a randomized controlled open-label study. J Clin Psychiatry. 2012;73(2):216-23. PMID: 21672497.

20. Karagianis J, Grossman L, Landry J, et al. A randomized controlled trial of the effect of sublingual orally disintegrating olanzapine versus oral olanzapine on body mass index: the PLATYPUS Study. Schizophr Res. 2009;113(1):41-8. PMID: 19535229.

21. Khazaal Y, Fresard E, Rabia S, et al. Cognitive behavioural therapy for weight gain associated with antipsychotic drugs. Schizophr Res. 2007;91(1-3):169-77. PMID: 17306507.

22. Kwon JS, Choi JS, Bahk WM, et al. Weight management program for treatment-emergent weight gain in olanzapine-treated patients with schizophrenia or schizoaffective disorder: A 12-week randomized controlled clinical trial. J Clin Psychiatry. 2006;67(4):547-53. PMID: 16669719.

23. Littrell KH, Hilligoss NM, Kirshner CD, et al. The effects of an educational intervention on antipsychotic-induced weight gain. J Nurs Scholarsh. 2003;35(3):237-41. PMID: 14562491.

24. Mauri M, Simoncini M, Castrogiovanni S, et al. A psychoeducational program for weight loss in patients who have experienced weight gain during antipsychotic treatment with olanzapine. Pharmacopsychiatry. 2008;41(1):17-23. PMID: 18203047.

25. McDonnell DP, Kryzhanovskaya LA, Zhao F, et al. Comparison of metabolic changes in patients with schizophrenia during randomized treatment with intramuscular olanzapine long-acting injection versus oral olanzapine. Hum Psychopharmacol. 2011;26(6):422-433. PMID: 21823172.

26. McElroy SL, Winstanley E, Mori N, et al. A randomized, placebo-controlled study of zonisamide to prevent olanzapine-associated weight gain. J Clin Psychopharmacol. 2012;32(2):165-72. PMID: 22367654.

27. McKibbin CL, Patterson TL, Norman G, et al. A lifestyle intervention for older schizophrenia patients with diabetes mellitus: a randomized controlled trial. Schizophr Res. 2006;86(1-3):36-44. PMID: 16842977.

28. Narula PK, Rehan HS, Unni KE, et al. Topiramate for prevention of olanzapine associated weight gain and metabolic dysfunction in schizophrenia: a double-blind, placebo-controlled trial. Schizophr Res. 2010;118(1-3):218-23. PMID: 20207521.

29. Newcomer JW, Campos JA, Marcus RN, et al. A multicenter, randomized, double-blind study of the effects of aripiprazole in overweight subjects with schizophrenia or schizoaffective disorder switched from olanzapine. J Clin Psychiatry. 2008;69(7):1046-56. PMID: 18605811.

30. Nickel MK, Nickel C, Muehlbacher M, et al. Influence of topiramate on olanzapine-related adiposity in women: a random, double-blind, placebo-controlled study. J Clin Psychopharmacol. 2005;25(3):211-7. PMID: 15876898.

31. Skrinar GS, Huxley NA, Hutchinson DS, et al. The role of a fitness intervention on people with serious psychiatric disabilities. Psychiatr Rehabil J. 2005;29(2):122-7. PMID: 16268007.

32. Stroup TS, McEvoy JP, Ring KD, et al. A randomized trial examining the effectiveness of switching from olanzapine, quetiapine, or risperidone to aripiprazole to reduce metabolic risk: comparison of antipsychotics for metabolic problems (CAMP). Am J Psychiatry. 2011;168(9):947-56. PMID: 21768610.

33. Wang M, Tong JH, Zhu G, et al. Metformin for treatment of antipsychotic-induced weight gain: a randomized, placebo-controlled study. Schizophr Res. 2012;138(1):54-7. PMID: 22398127.

34. Wu RR, Zhao JP, Jin H, et al. Lifestyle intervention and metformin for treatment of antipsychotic-induced weight gain: a randomized controlled trial. JAMA. 2008;299(2):185-93. PMID: 18182600.

35. Wu RR, Jin H, Gao K, et al. Metformin for Treatment of Antipsychotic-Induced Amenorrhea and Weight Gain in Women With First-Episode Schizophrenia: A Double-Blind, Randomized, Placebo-Controlled Study. Am J Psychiatry. 2012. PMID: 22711171.